Outcome Measures in
Alzheimer's Disease

Cover figure courtesy of Jeffrey L Cummings (see Figure 4.4, Page 48).

Outcome Measures in Alzheimer's Disease

Edited by

Ian G McKeith

With

Jeffrey L Cummings
Richard J Harvey
Simon Lovestone
David G Wilkinson

MARTIN DUNITZ

© Martin Dunitz Ltd 1999

First published in the United Kingdom in 1999 by

Martin Dunitz Ltd
The Livery House
7–9 Pratt Street
London NW1 0AE

A CIP record for this book is available from the British Library.

ISBN 1-85317-745-8

Distributed in the United States by:
Blackwell Science Inc.
Commerce Place, 350 Main Street
Malden, MA 02148, USA
Tel: 1-800-215-1000

Distributed in Canada by:
Login Brothers Book Company
324 Salteaux Crescent
Winnipeg, Manitoba, R3J 3T2
Canada
Tel: 204-224-4068

Distributed in Brazil by:
Ernesto Reichmann Distribuidora de Livros, Ltda
Rua Coronel Marques 335, Tatuape 03440-000
Sao Paulo,
Brazil

Composition by Scribe Design, Gillingham, Kent, UK
Printed and bound in Italy by Printer Trento srl.

Contents

Contributors   vii

Introduction   ix

1. Cognitive function   1
    Ian G McKeith

2. Global function   15
    Richard J Harvey

3. Activities of daily living   27
    Simon Lovestone

4. Neuropsychiatric symptoms   37
    Jeffrey L Cummings

5. Quality of life   51
    Caroline E Selai and Richard J Harvey

6. Caregiver burden   63
    David G Wilkinson and Cathey Dukes

Index   73

Contributors

Jeffrey L Cummings MD
Departments of Neurology and Psychiatry &
Behavioral Sciences
UCLA School of Medicine
Los Angeles, USA

Cathey Dukes MBChB MRCPsych
Thornhill Research Unit
Moorgreen Hospital
Southampton, UK

Richard J Harvey MD MRCPsych
Dementia Research Group
Institute of Neurology
The National Hospital for Neurology
and Neurosurgery
London, UK

Simon Lovestone MPhil MRCPsych PhD
Institute of Psychiatry
London, UK

Ian G McKeith MD FRCPsych
Institute for the Health of the Elderly
Newcastle General Hospital
Newcastle-upon-Tyne, UK

Caroline E Selai MSc
Raymond Way Neuropsychiatry
Research Group
Institute of Neurology
The National Hospital for Neurology
and Neurosurgery
London, UK

David G Wilkinson MBChB MRCGP
FRCPsych
Thornhill Research Unit
Moorgreen Hospital
Southampton, UK

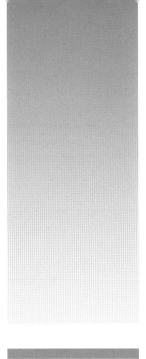

Introduction

Alzheimer's disease—no longer untreatable

Alzheimer's disease (AD) is now widely acknowledged as the most common cause of dementia with a prevalence of 30% or more in people over the age of 85 years. Definitions of AD generally refer to it as being progressive and irreversible, which has promoted a surrounding air of therapeutic nihilism. Its effects upon sufferers and carers certainly can be devastating, imposing heavy demands upon personal, health, social and financial resources. One response to the increasing public concern about AD has been a progressive increase in biomedical and psychosocial research into the condition during the last two decades. As a consequence of this activity, we now have accurate estimates of the prevalence and incidence of AD in the population, the risk doubling every 4-5 years over the age of 65. The events leading to selective neuronal degeneration in AD are beginning to be understood at a molecular level and an increasing number of causative and relative risk genes have been identified. Clinicians with appropriate training and experience can now diagnose AD with an accuracy of 85–90%, confirmed by brain tissue examination at autopsy. The first generation of rationally based, anti-Alzheimer drug treatments have recently reached clinical practice, in the form of cholinesterase inhibitors which exert their effects by increasing the availability of acetyl- and/or butyl-choline in the central nervous system. Although the symptomatic effects of these new drugs are generally modest, they represent the beginning of a new era in the management of AD. They have imbued an optimism that we will eventually move to very early or pre-symptomatic diagnosis, followed by intervention with agents which are able to delay significantly, or even prevent, disease onset and progression.

Which symptoms of AD do we need to treat?

In 1907, when Dr Alois Alzheimer described a 51-year-old woman with progressive dementia, he reported upon a wide range of clinical manifestations of what later came to be called 'Alzheimer's disease'. These included intellectual impairments which were sufficiently severe to impair her capacity for self care, in addition to which she suffered early and prominent delusions and hallucinations which led to profound agitation and the need for restraint and institutional care (Maurer et al 1997). Many subsequent reports have confirmed that the consequences of neuronal loss and neurotransmitter deficits in AD are manifest in a wide range of clinical symptoms. Alzheimer's disease is not simply a disease of intellectual decline and memory failure—psychiatric features such as anxiety, depression, hallucinations, delusions, and sleep and appetite disturbance are frequently prominent and these impact directly upon the sufferer's ability to carry out normal social and occupational functions. It is usually the behavioural disturbances and functional disabilities associated with AD which carers find most stressful and which may eventually prompt referral to specialist services for additional support and treatment, including requests for institutional care.

In deciding which symptoms of AD we need to treat in a particular patient, it is therefore essential to know the following:

- Which of the wide ranging manifestations of AD are present?
- How distressing or trouble-some are these different symptoms and disabilities to the sufferer and carer?
- Which (if any) are likely to respond to the treatments currently available?

Outcome measures in AD

By the time that AD is clinically apparent, many interconnected brain structures and systems are severely compromised. Alzheimer's disease is therefore usually regarded as producing a global dysfunction of intellect and behaviour. Any attempt to subdivide the symptomatology of AD into separate components might be criticized on the grounds that the different manifestations are intimately interrelated, eg, the failure to recognize other people and therefore to behave aggressively towards them, may be secondary to impaired visual perception and

deficits in semantic memory. Severe anxiety may be an understandable response to the patient's fear that their spouse has abandoned them, because they have simply forgotten that the other person is in the next room. In clinical practice, however, there is much to commend identifying four principal domains affected by AD, namely:

- Cognition
- Global functioning
- Activities of daily living
- Neuropsychiatric features

Each of these domains is associated with specific methods of assessment and scales for quantification and measurement of change over time. Other measurable dimensions of AD are quality of life and caregiver burden, both important determinants of care needs and outcome.

Ian McKeith
Newcastle, UK, 1999

Reference

Maurer K, Volk S, Gerbaldo H (1997) Auguste D and Alzheimer's disease. *Lancet* **349**:1546–9.

Cognitive function

Clinical definitions of dementia, particularly those for Alzheimer's disease, emphasize the primacy of cognitive (intellectual) decline. DSM-IV, ICD-10, and NINCDS-ADRDA criteria all require memory failure to be present (**Table 1.1**), but there is less unanimity about the precise characteristics of other cognitive deficits (Cummings and Khachaturian 1996).

Patients with AD typically present with occasional failure of episodic memory (memory for events) which progressively becomes more severe and persistent according to Ribot's Law (last in, first out). Other memory functions also become involved as the pathological disease progresses from limbic structures to the neocortex, eg, semantic memory which contains meaning and knowledge about objects, words, facts, concepts and their relationships. As a consequence patients experience language difficulties and misidentify their environment, and people and objects within it. Implicit (procedural) memory, which enables us to carry out skills which have previously been

Table 1.1
Cognitive deficits in Alzheimer's disease. ICD-10, DSM IV and NINCDS-ADRDA criteria compared.
(Adapted from Cummings and Khachaturian 1996)

	ICD-10	DSM IV	NINCDS/ADRDA probable AD
Declining memory	+	+	+
At least one of:			
'Non-memory' intellectual impairment	+	+	+
Impaired thinking	+	–	–
Aphasia, apraxia, agnosia, or impaired executive function	–	+	–
Decline from previous level	+	+	+
Insidious onset	+	+	–
Slow deterioration	+	–	–
Continuing deterioration	–	+	–
Deficits not limited to delirious period	+	+	+

overlearned and performed without consciousness awareness, eg, using a knife and fork, is generally spared until the late stages of AD.

Whilst memory impairments are undoubtedly common in AD, they represent only one aspect of a much wider range of cognitive deficits, some of which may be functionally far more disabling. These include attentional.

deficits, language disorders, visuospatial difficulties, dyspraxias and executive dysfunction. Each of these should be assessed in even the most basic cognitive examination.

Objectives of assessment

Cognitive function may be assessed for a variety of overlapping reasons which are listed in **Table 1.2**.

Table 1.2
Possible objectives of cognitive assessment in a patient with suspected or established dementia.

Screening
Confirmation of diagnosis
Subtype diagnosis
Severity
Rate of progression

Screening programmes aim to identify individuals whose cognitive performance is less than that predicted for age, education and social class. Cognitive screening tools are not sufficient in themselves to diagnose dementia. Low scores may be due to dementia delirium, depression, physical ill health, low educational status, sensory impairments or frequently, a combination of these.

Confirmation of diagnosis of dementia requires a history of decline from the previous level of cognitive performance. This may be obvious in moderately affected individuals, for example, a retired teacher who is now unable to remember which day of the week it is. In patients with early disease, cognitive decline may be hard to identify and estimates of previous intellectual functioning are required for comparison with the current level of cognitive performance. Premorbid IQ is typically assessed using tests such as the National Adult Reading Test (NART), which requires subjects to read aloud correctly from a list containing words which range from the common to the obscure. It is not necessary to know the meaning of the words (which would be a test of semantic memory) but simply to pronounce them correctly, thereby indicating previous exposure and familiarity.

The profile of cognitive impairments may be a useful indicator of the underlying disease process and **subtype diagnosis**. Alzheimer's disease usually presents with episodic memory impairment followed later by executive dysfunction, dysphasia and dyspraxia. Dementia with Lewy bodies (DLB; McKeith et al 1996), typically has prominent attentional deficits with relative preservation of episodic memory, especially in the early stages. Executive dysfunction and visuospatial impairments may be disproportionately severe in DLB. Focal cognitive impairments, eg, a non-fluent expressive dysphasia accompanied by focal neurological deficits may occur in vascular dementia (VaD) which is caused by multiple infarcts. Progressive cerebral ischaemia due to small vessel disease may, however, lack this pattern (Roman et al 1993). Patients with fronto-temporal dementia (FTD; Snowdon et al 1996) may show early and severe impairment of semantic memory and language and perform poorly on mental tasks requiring a degree of effort such as verbal fluency or the Trailmaking test.

Severity of impairment on cognitive testing is generally expressed as a single score when brief procedures are used. More complex batteries additionally allow sub-scores to be expressed for different aspects of cognition, eg, memory, language and praxis.

Retesting at 6–12 monthly intervals allows **rate of progression** to be calculated and compared with normative data. Patients with AD typically decline by 10–15% of maximum test score per annum, but there is a high degree of variability between patients, some individuals deteriorating rapidly, with others showing little or no change. The amount of change is partly dependent upon the severity of their dementia at baseline assessment. Patients with mild impairment generally show less change over the following year than more severely impaired patients. This reflects more upon the psychometric properties

of most cognitive tests (see below— ceiling and floor effects), than upon the underlying pathological processes. For an individual patient with AD the rate of cognitive decline over the previous 12 months may be used as a very approximate guide to the anticipated deterioration over the coming year.

Performance on cognitive testing is only moderately correlated with measures of functional disability, global functioning and the presence of neuropsychiatric features. Cognitive test scores should therefore not be used in isolation as an expression of severity of dementia. This is particularly important when assessing an AD patient's response to treatment. Global, behavioural and activity of daily living (ADL) functions may change significantly, for better or worse, without a corresponding change in cognitive performance (and vice versa).

Cognitive symptoms to be examined

Cognitive assessment should consist of a brief examination of the items listed in **Table 1.3**. Testing should be done within the context of a comprehensive mental state examination which records the presence or absence or behavioural

Table 1.3
Items which should be routinely examined during cognitive assessment. Those marked* are usually incorporated within simple cognitive screening instruments, eg, MMSE. Other items need to be judged within a comprehensive mental state examination.

> *Previous intellectual performance*
> *Mood*
> *Cooperation/motivation*
> *Attention**
> *Orientation**
> *Memory**
> *Language**
> *Visuospatial/constructional abilities**
> *Calculation**
> *Abstract thinking*
> *Insight*

disturbance, the level of cooperation and the degree of insight. Affective status should always be evaluated since anxiety and depression may have a major impact on cognitive performance.

Tools used

A list of selected cognitive test procedures is given in **Tables 1.4** and **1.5**.

Simple tools

Short, easily administered tests suitable for screening large numbers of elderly people in primary care or geriatric

Table 1.4
Simple cognitive tests suitable for screening and measuring overall severity of cognitive impairment in AD.

Test functions name	Range (worst to best)	Average annual rate of decline (points/year)	Cognitive tested
Blessed Information, Memory, Concentration Test (BIMC)	0-37	3–4	Orientation, attention, recent and long-term memory (recall)
Mini Mental State Examination (MMSE)	0–30	2–4	Orientation, recent and long-term memory (recall), naming, comprehension, praxis, calculation
Syndrome Kurztest (SKT)	27–0	2–4	Recall and recognition memory, naming, attention, praxis

medicine practice, or for repeated use, include the Blessed Information, Memory and Concentration test (BIMC; Blessed et al 1968), the Mini Mental State Examination (MMSE; Folstein et al 1975) and the Syndrome Kurztest (SKT; Erigkeit 1989). The BIMC tests attention, orientation, and short- and long-term memory. These are supplemented in the MMSE by tests of language, ability to read, write and draw. The MMSE which is easily administered in less than 10 minutes is the most widely used cognitive assessment procedure. A score of 23 or less out of 30 is associated with a significantly increased probability of a diagnosis of dementia. SKT which is widely used in German-speaking countries, consists of a series of timed performance tasks which predominantly test attention and memory.

Complex tools

These fall into two main types. Tests like the Cambridge Cognitive Examination (CAMCOG; Roth et al 1986) and the Mattis Dementia Rating Scale (DRS; Mattis 1976) are essentially extended screening instruments, suitable for use by clinicians. These scales briefly examine a wider range of cognitive functions, the results of which can still be expressed by a single total score. Much more extensive neuropsychological test batteries, eg, the Kendrick Test Battery (Kendrick et al 1979) are usually administered and interpreted by expert neuropsychologists and may require several testing sessions for completion (3–4 hours in total). Different components may be incorporated into such batteries depending upon the particular aspects of cognition to be explored in depth.

The cognitive section of the Alzheimer's Disease Assessment Scale (ADAS-COG; Mohs and Cohen 1988) falls somewhere between these two categories of complex testing. It may take up to an hour to administer and although it is not generally used in routine clinical practice, it has been accepted as the most commonly used neuropsychological outcome measure for anti-dementia drug trials. The subtests within ADAS-COG are listed in **Table 1.5**. It is worth noting that some important aspects of cognition are not assessed with ADAS-COG, these include working memory, delayed recall, attention, agnosia and executive function.

Pros and cons

The relative merits of different test procedures depend upon the precise

Table 1.5
More complex cognitive tests suitable for confirmation of a diagnosis of dementia and for profiling diagnostic subtypes including AD. CAMCOG and ADAS have high ceiling effects whereas DRS and SIB have low floor effects, making combinations of these tests sensitive across a wide range of severity of AD

Test functions name	Range (worst to best)	Average annual rate of decline (points/year)	Cognitive tested
Cambridge Cognitive Examination (CAMCOG)	0–107	10–12	Memory (recall and recognition), orientation, attention, praxis, perception, language, calculation, abstract thinking
Alzheimer's Disease Assessment Scale (ADAS-COG)	70–0	7–9	Memory (recall and recognition), orientation, language, praxis
Mattis Dementia Rating Scale (DRS)	0–144	10–12	Attention, perseveration, memory (recall), praxis, abstract thinking
Severe Impairment Battery (SIB)	0–100	N/A	Memory, orientation, attention, language, praxis, visuospatial ability, social interaction

objectives of the assessment. The ideal screening instrument should contain memory and non-memory items, be acceptable to demented and non-demented subjects alike, achieve high inter-rater reliability, be quick to administer, and have widely available normative data. The MMSE fulfils most of these requirements, although slight variations in administration and interpretation of responses can lead to differences of several points in total scores. Extended versions (CAMCOG, DRS) are most suitable for use in dementia assessment services (geriatric medicine, old age psychiatry and neurology) but require properly trained raters to spend significant amounts of time engaged in testing. Day hospital and community nurses, and psychology assistants often administer these procedures. The more complex test batteries should be administered by expert raters under highly standardized conditions.

Floor and ceiling effects are particularly problematic. Both simple and complex tools have generally been designed to have maximum sensitivity to change in the mild to moderate stages of AD. Simple instruments are insensitive to the earliest stages of cognitive decline and patients who complain of significant intellectual deterioration may score at, or close to, 100% on the MMSE. Conversely, patients with moderate to severe AD may be barely able to achieve any score on most cognitive tests (a floor effect), their difficulties being compounded by an inability to understand test instructions or to verbalize their responses. The Severe Impairment Battery (SIB; Panisset et al 1994) and Test for Severe Impairment (Albert and Cohen 1992) have been specifically developed to address the problem of floor effects. Global, neuropsychiatric and ADL scales are typically more relevant and measurable indicators of performance in the later stages of AD.

Evaluation of current therapies

Regulatory authorities in North America and Europe require putative anti-dementia drugs to show effects upon cognition. The reasons for this are two-fold. First, memory failure is central to all current definitions of dementia and Alzheimer's disease, therefore a treatment which improves memory carries a high face validity. Second, most currently available treatments affect cholinergic neurotransmission, and cholinergic deficits in post-mortem brain tissue, have been correlated with ante-mortem memory performance.

The ADAS-COG has generally been adopted as the 'gold standard' measure of cognition in anti-dementia drug trials. ADAS-COG is familiar to clinical investigators, pharmaceutical companies and regulatory bodies, but is not well known by most clinicians, who therefore experience difficulty in interpreting clinical trial data. The most often quoted cognitive outcome measure in anti-dementia trials is the change in ADAS-COG scores (Δ ADAS-COG) before and after 26 weeks of treatment. The difference between Δ ADAS-COG scores for placebo and active drug-treated patients is taken as a measure of effect size. **Figure 1.1** shows typical data from a hypothetical trial A. There is a statistically significant difference between active and placebo groups at week 26 which in this case amounts to an absolute difference of

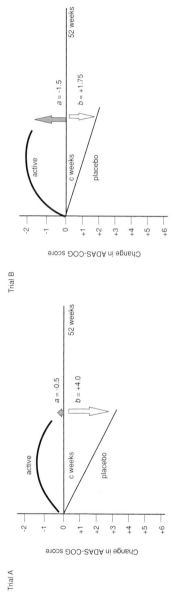

Trial A

Change in ADAS-COG score

active

$a = -0.5$

$b = +4.0$

c weeks

52 weeks

placebo

Difference in ADAS-COG test score at week 26 = $(a - b)$ = 4.5 points
Annualized rate of placebo decline = $2b$ = 8.0 points
Disease progression equivalent = $\dfrac{(a - b)}{2b}$ = 0.56 years = 6.8 months

Trial B

Change in ADAS-COG score

active

$a = -1.5$

$b = +1.75$

c weeks

52 weeks

placebo

Difference in ADAS-COG test score at week 26 = $(a - b)$ = 3.25 points
Annualized rate of placebo decline = $2b$ = 3.5 points
Disease progression equivalent = $\dfrac{(a - b)}{2b}$ = 0.93 years = 11.2 months

Figures 1.1 and 1.2
Trials A and B illustrate two different ways of estimating cognitive effects of anti-dementia drugs. The difference in ADAS-COG test scores between drug and placebo groups is greater in trial A (4.5 points) than in trial B (3.25 points). However, when placebo deterioration rates are accounted for, the effect size expressed as disease progression is greater in trial B (11.3 months) than in trial A (6.8 months).

Table 1.6
Effect sizes of anti-AD drugs in selected trials, expressed as change in ADAS-COG scores and as disease progression equivalents. Apparent differences between drugs probably reflects variation between study populations and true differences in efficacy cannot reliably be inferred.

Drug name and daily dose	Change in ADAS-COG (active vs placebo)	Disease progression equivalent
Tacrine 120/60 mg (Knapp et al 1994)	5.3 points at 26 weeks	12.7 months
Donepezil 10 mg (Rogers et al 1998)	2.9 points at 24 weeks	8.9 months
Rivastigmine 6–12 mg (Corey-Bloom et al 1998)	3.8 points at 26 weeks	5.6 months
Metrifonate 30–60 mg (Cummings et al 1998)	2.9 points at 12 weeks	13.4 months
Ginkgo biloba 120 mg (Le Bars et al 1997)	1.7 points at 52 weeks	13.6 months

4.5 ADAS-COG points. How can the clinical significance of this symptomatic treatment effect be judged? It has been suggested that one method is to convert any improvement in cognitive score into a period of time for deterioration of a similar magnitude to occur as part of a natural disease progression (Rogers et al 1998). Initially such calculations were based on reports that typical AD patients deteriorate an average of 9 points per annum. Thus for a trial showing an active drug/placebo difference of 4.5 points the treatment effect could be regarded as equivalent to the reversal of 6 months worth of disease progression. This is a reasonable approximation for trial A. **Figure 1.2** shows trial B which is of similar design, but in which the active drug/placebo difference at 26 weeks (*a–b*) is only 3.25 points—a treatment effect which apparently is less than trial A. Closer inspection of **Figure 1.2** shows, however, that the placebo group deteriorated by only 1.75 points over 6 months, equivalent to 3.5 points per annum. If the disease progression equivalent of this treatment effect is calculated using the formula $(a-b)/2b$, ie, ADAS-COG effect divided by the annualized rate of placebo decline in the given study, the effect size in trial A is $4.5/8 = 0.56$ years (6.8 months disease reversal) and in trial B is $3.25/3.5 = 0.93$ years (11.2 months).

Table 1.6 summarizes effect sizes for a variety of anti-dementia medications, expressing these both as Δ ADAS-COG scores and as disease progression equivalents. It is immediately apparent that the two parameters are not well correlated. The disease progression equivalent calculation is much more dependent on the placebo deterioration rate (b in Figure 1.1) than it is upon improvement over baseline (a). Since clinical trials have all been conducted in independent populations and by different investigators, it is probably unwise to compare either Δ ADAS-COG or disease progression equivalents as a basis for measuring different drugs against each other.

Future developments in assessing symptoms

Cognitive outcome measures are only one part of assessing the impairments of dementia, rates of decline and response to treatment. Future refinements might include the following:

- Improving the administration of simple cognitive screening tests by standardized guidelines, training and supervision.
- Ensuring that test procedures in routine clinical use are sufficiently comprehensive to assess the broad range of cognitive deficits of AD.
- Floor and ceiling effects need to be addressed. Computer-based neuropsychological test batteries (COGDRAS; Simpson et al 1991; CANTAB; Morris et al 1987) are able not only to detect small changes at high levels of performance but also to measure previously unassessed aspects of cognitive function including motor and cognitive response latency. The Severe Impairment Battery and Test for Severe Impairment both collect useful cognitive data in the later stages.
- Methods of estimating and comparing cognitive outcomes in anti-dementia drug trials need to be further refined and widely disseminated.

References

Albert M, Cohen C (1992) The test for severe impairment: an instrument for the assessment of patients with severe cognitive dysfunction. *J Am Geriatr Soc* **40**:449–53.

Blessed G, Tomlinson BE, Roth M (1968) The association between quantitative measures of dementia and senile change in the cerebral gray matter of elderly subjects. *Br J Psychiatry* **114**:797–811.

Corey-Bloom J, Anand R, Veach J, for the ENA 713 B352 Study Group (1998) A randomized trial evaluating the efficacy and safety of ENA 713 (rivastigmine tartrate), a new acetylcholinesterase inhibitor, in patients with mild to moderately severe Alzheimer's disease. *Int J Geriat Psychopharmacol* **1**:55–65.

Cummings JC, Khachaturian Z (1996) Definitions and diagnostic criteria. In: Gauthier S (ed.) *Clinical Diagnosis and Management of Alzheimer's Disease*. Martin Dunitz, London: 3–15.

Cummings JL, Cyrus PA, Mas J et al and the Metrifonate Study Group (1998) Metrifonate treatment of the cognitive deficits of Alzheimer's disease. *Neurology* **50**:1214–21.

Erigkeit H (1989) The SKT – a short cognitive performance test as an instrument for the assessment of clinical efficacy of cognition enhancers. In: Bergener M and Reisberg B (eds), *Diagnosis and Treatment of Senile Dementia*. Springer-Verlag, Berlin: 164–74.

Folstein MF, Folstein SE, McHugh PR (1975) Mini-mental state. A practical method for grading the cognitive state of patients for the clinician. *J Psychiat Res* **12**:189–98.

Kendrick DC, Gibson AJ, Moyes CA (1979) The revised Kendrick Battery: clinical studies. *Br J Clin Psychol* **18**:329–40.

Knapp MJ, Knopman DS, Solomon PR (1994) A 30 week randomised controlled trial of high-dose tacrine in patients with Alzheimer's disease. *JAMA* **271**:985–91.

Le Bars PL, Katz MM, Berman N et al (1997) A placebo-controlled, double-blind, randomized trial of an extract of Ginkgo biloba for dementia. North American EGb Study Group *JAMA* **278**:1327–32.

McKeith IG, Galasko D, Kosaka K et al (1996) Consensus guidelines for the clinical and pathologic diagnosis of dementia with Lewy bodies (DLB): report of the consortium on DLB international workshop. *Neurology* **47**:1113–24.

Mattis S (1976) Mental status examination for organic mental syndrome in the elderly patient. In: Bellack R and Karasu B (eds), *Geriatric Psychiatry*. Grune and Stratton, New York: 77–121.

Mohs RC, Cohen L (1988) Alzheimer's Disease Assessment Scale (ADAS). *Psychopharmacol Bull* **24**:627–8.

Morris R, Evenden J, Sahakian B, Robbins T (1987) Computer aided assessment of dementia. In: Stahl S, Iversen S and Goodman E (eds), *Cognitive Neurochemistry* Oxford University Press, Oxford: 21–36.

Panisset M, Roudier M, Saxton J, Boller F (1994) Severe impairment battery. A neuropsychological test for severely demented patients. *Arch Neurol* **51**:41–6.

Rogers SL, Farlow MR, Doody RS et al and the Donepezil Study Group (1998) A 24 week double blind, placebo-controlled trial of donepezil in patients with Alzheimer's disease. *Neurology* **50**:136–45.

Roman G, Tatemichi TK, Erkinjuntti T and the NINDS-AIREN Workgroup (1993) Vascular dementia: diagnostic criteria for research studies. Report of the NINDS-AIREN International Workshop. *Neurology* **43**:250–60.

Roth M, Tym E, Mountjoy CQ et al (1986) CAMDEX: A standard instrument for the diagnosis of mental disorder in the elderly with special reference to the early detection of dementia. *Br J Psychiat* **149**:698–709.

Simpson PM, Surmon DJ, Wesnes KA, Wilcock CG (1991) The Cognitive Drug Research computerised assessment system for demented patients: a validation study. *Int J Geriatr Psychiat* **6**:95–102.

Snowdon JS, Neary D, Mann DMA (1996) *Fronto-temporal Lobar Degeneration: Fronto-temporal Dementia, Progressive Aphasia, Semantic Dementia.* Churchill Livingstone, Edinburgh.

Global function

2

Objectives of the assessment

An assessment of global function is one of the primary outcome measures upon which the effects of an anti-dementia drug are assessed. The intention of the assessment is to obtain a rating of the patient made by someone experienced in the assessment of dementia taking into account information collected from a wide-ranging interview. Global ratings are intended to provide an informative index of change that cannot be solely obtained from quantitative assessment measures such as mental status examinations. There are three types of global assessment commonly used in clinical trials: disease staging measures; absolute global severity assessments; and clinical global change ratings.

Disease staging measures are based on semi-structured assessments of the patient with information from the caregiver and other sources. The patient is then placed on the spectrum of disease severity defined by

	Global change scale		Global severity scale
1	➡	Very much improved	➡	Normal, not ill at all
2	➡	Much improved	➡	Borderline mentally ill
3	➡	Minimally improved	➡	Mildly ill
4	➡	No change	➡	Moderately ill
5	➡	Minimally worse	➡	Markedly ill
6	➡	Much worse	➡	Severely ill
7	➡	Very much worse	➡	Among the most extremely ill

Figure 2.1
The seven-point global rating

the scale, according to specific guidelines. Staging measures are very useful for selecting patients for a clinical trial, but they are unsuitable for use as primary outcomes in trials of less than 1–2 years duration; this is because over shorter periods patients naturally tend not to move from one severity category to another. This property makes them stable and reliable as staging measures, but insensitive to the small effects on disease severity likely to be seen with current anti-dementia drugs.

Absolute global severity assessments capture the overall severity of a patient's illness by reference to the full spectrum of disease severity. From this baseline, the global change measure is intended to capture the extent of improvement or deterioration in the patient which is perceived to have occurred by the clinician since the baseline severity assessment. At the beginning of the clinical trial, the clinician making the global rating assesses the patient to their own satisfaction and makes a global rating of disease severity on the seven-point scale. This rating, together with the experience and understanding of the patient that the clinician has gained, acts as a baseline against which subsequent ratings of change are made. At subsequent assessments the clinician making the global rating is expected to grade the patient on a seven-point scale of change (**Figure 2.1**), by reference on

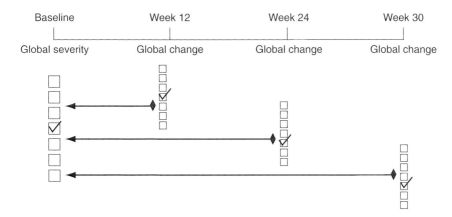

Figure 2.2
Global assessment of change is always made by reference to the baseline assessment of global severity

each occasion to the baseline severity assessment (**Figure 2.2**).

The validity and reliability of global measures relies heavily on the clinician's skills, training, and previous experience. In a multi-centre clinical trial with 20–30 centres, there may be as many as 50 clinicians making global ratings. For such a subjective and unstructured assessment to be effective, investigator training and inter-rater reliability are critical. The various enhancements and developments of the global rating attempt to improve inter-rater reliability principally by structuring and standardizing the assessment that forms the basis of the rating. The subjective and personal nature of the global rating means that it is imperative that the same clinician makes the rating on each occasion for a particular patient.

Tools used

Disease staging measures

Clinical dementia rating (CDR) (Berg 1988)

The CDR is a staging measure based on a six-point scale. The rating is based on a structured interview with the carer followed by a structured interview with and assessment of the patient. Ratings from 0 to 3, including a 0.5 (questionable) value, are made in the domains of: memory; orientation; judgement and problem solving; community affairs; home and hobbies; and personal care.

The rating from each domain can then either be summed to give the CDR-SB (Sum of Boxes) score, or an algorithm weighted on the memory domain can be used to give a 0–3 score, with additional profound (4) and terminal (5) scores available.

Global deterioration scale (GDS) (Reisberg et al 1982)

The GDS is a seven-point severity staging measure. The rating is made on the basis of interviews with the patient and caregiver covering each stage of the scale from the mildest to the most severe in turn. As the interview progresses to increasingly severe deficits a point will be reached were deficits are no longer reported. The highest incapacity stage then forms the rating of the GDS.

Functional assessment staging (FAST) (Reisberg 1988)

The FAST incorporates the GDS but further subdivides GDS stages 6 (moderate to severe) and 7 (severe) into 10 substages. The same hierarchical method of identifying deficits and placing patients into their highest incapacity rating is used to obtain the FAST score.

Table 2.1 summarizes the interrelationship between the three staging measures.

Clinical global measures

CGIS/CGIC (clinical global impression of severity/change) (Guy 1976)

This is the global assessment most commonly used in non-dementia psychopharmacological trials. There are minimal instructions or guidelines and it primarily requires a skilled clinician to make a judgement of severity or change. The rating is based on the clinician's experience taking all factors into account, irrespective of whether or not the rater believes the effect is due to the drug. The rater may or may not interview the patient or carer, access other sources of information, and have access to cognitive tests.

A considerably experienced physician is needed to make the assessment, although they do not necessarily need to see the patient. Moreover the assessment is easily biased and can be unblinded if the physician has access to details of adverse events. For this reason the CGIC has not been used in anti-dementia studies since the early 1990s.

CIBIS/CIBIC (clinicians interview-based impression of severity/change) (Leber 1990)

The basis of the CIBIS/CIBIC is outlined by the US Food and Drug Administration (FDA) in their guidelines on evaluation

Table 2.1
Comparison of the CDR, GDS and FAST.

Clinical disease stage	Estimated MMSE score	CDR stage	GDS stage	FAST stage
Normal	30	0	1	1
Forgetfulness of old age			2	2
Mild memory impairment/incipient/ questionable dementia		0.5	3	3
Mild dementia	24		4	4
Moderate dementia	19	1	5	5
Moderate-severe dementia	14	2	6	6a
				6b
	10			6c
		3		6d
	5			6e
Severe dementia	2	4	7	7a
	0			7b
				7c
				7d
		5		7e
				7f

of anti-dementia drugs (Leber 1990). The rationale of the assessment is that a clinically meaningful anti-dementia drug effect should be detectable by a clinician interviewing the patient in isolation from other sources of information including the caregiver. On this basis, any change rated by the clinician must be clinically meaningful.

As with the CGIC, the CIBIS/CIBIC has minimal guidelines, and thus suffers from high inter-rater variability, and from the concern that excluding the caregiver from the assessment is unnatural in clinical practice and may bias any rating.

Parke-Davis CIBIC (Knopman et al 1994; Schneider and Olin 1997)

This assessment involves a thorough baseline interview with both patient and caregiver covering eight specific domains (history, patient strengths and weaknesses, language, behaviour, motivation, activities of daily living, other areas of importance). The assessment makes use of worksheets that encourage standardization, and provide a source of notes for the rater to refer back to on subsequent assessments. At follow-up, the patient in interviewed alone and a change in the rating is made.

Sandoz/New York University CIBIC-plus (NYU CIBIC-plus) (Reisberg and Ferris 1994)

The term CIBIC-plus refers to global assessments that require information from the patient *plus* caregiver to make each rating. The NYU CIBIC-plus is based on a fully structured interview with the patient and caregiver that ensures a comprehensive assessment of cognition, behaviour, and functioning by a clinician blind to the psychometric test scores. The rating of change is made on the usual seven-point scale, except that standardized guidelines for assessing change are given (**Table 2.2**).

Alzheimer's disease co-operative study — clinical global impression of change (ADCS–CGIC) (Schneider et al 1997)

The ADCS-CGIC was designed by obtaining clinicians' opinions and adapting existing instruments. The rating is based upon an organized but unstructured interview format which expects the rater to assess various domains including memory, language, orientation, praxis, mood, abnormal behaviour, and activities of daily living.

Unlike the fully structured NYU-CIBIC where every patient is assessed in the same way, in the ADCS-CGIC the rater is expected to make up his or her own assessments for each domain. The final rating incorporates information from both the patient and caregiver, and is therefore a CIBIC+. It is only the second global measure to have had a formal validation study published.

Other versions of the CIBIC+

Every regulatory quality anti-dementia drug trial must include a global rating. It has become commonplace for pharmaceutical companies to develop or adapt their own versions of the CIBIC+ in consultation with the FDA and other regulators. In many cases a validation of the specific format of the instrument is either not published, or has not been performed and some caution is therefore required in their interpretation. In particular, to date, there have been no cross-validation studies comparing different forms of the CIBIC, and this is another reason why extreme care is needed in any attempt to compare trials of one drug with another.

Changes on the global rating in a 6-month clinical trial will tend to be very small. **Figure 2.3** combines validation data from the ADCS-CGIC (Schneider et al 1997)

Table 2.2
Global rating guidelines.

Rating	Sandoz/NYU-CIBIC-plus Guideline (although final global rating remains a matter of clinical judgement)	ADCS-CGIC Guideline
1 point (minimal) change	There should be a 'detectable' change in the patient	Small change in one domain
2 points (moderate) change	The degree of change should be 'clearly apparent'	Definite change in one domain or small change in more than one domain.
3 points (marked) change	The change in the patient should be considered 'dramatic'	Definite change in more than one domain.

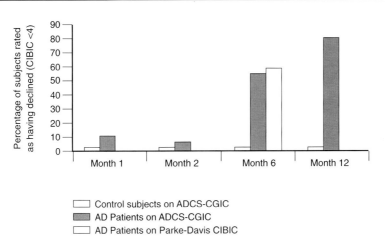

☐ Control subjects on ADCS-CGIC
▨ AD Patients on ADCS-CGIC
☐ AD Patients on Parke-Davis CIBIC

Figure 2.3
Changes on global ratings in untreated AD patients and control subjects

and the Parke-Davis CIBIC (Knopman et al 1994). The most notable feature is that after 6 months only approximately 60% of untreated patients with Alzheimer's disease will be rated to have changed (score <4).

Table 2.3
Evaluation of some current therapies on global function

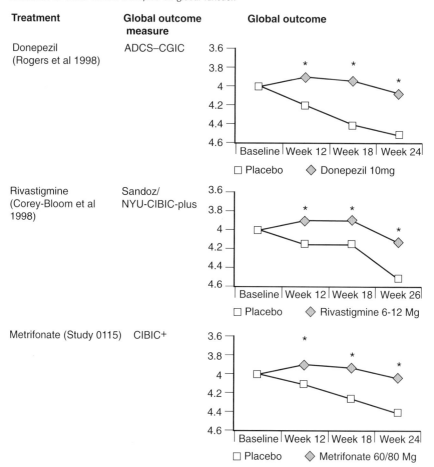

Treatment	Global outcome measure	Global outcome

Donepezil (Rogers et al 1998) — ADCS–CGIC

Baseline | Week 12 | Week 18 | Week 24
□ Placebo   ◇ Donepezil 10mg

Rivastigmine (Corey-Bloom et al 1998) — Sandoz/ NYU-CIBIC-plus

Baseline | Week 12 | Week 18 | Week 26
□ Placebo   ◇ Rivastigmine 6-12 Mg

Metrifonate (Study 0115) — CIBIC+

Baseline | Week 12 | Week 18 | Week 24
□ Placebo   ◇ Metrifonate 60/80 Mg

Evaluation of some current therapies on global function

Table 2.3 summarizes the type of global measures used, and the clinical trial outcome for a range of current therapies for Alzheimer's disease. Results have been presented on a uniform scale, although as studies

Treatment	Global outcome measure	Global outcome

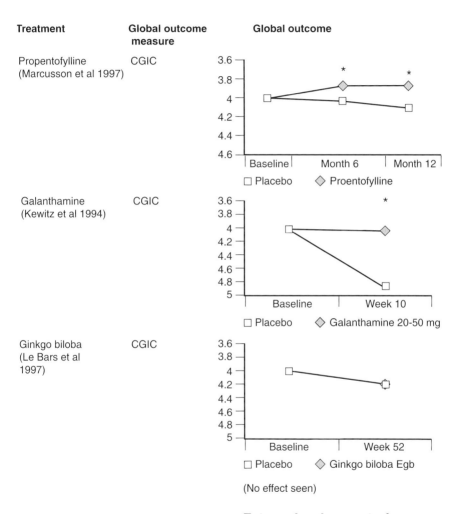

Propentofylline (Marcusson et al 1997) — CGIC
□ Placebo   ◇ Proentofylline

Galanthamine (Kewitz et al 1994) — CGIC
□ Placebo   ◇ Galanthamine 20-50 mg

Ginkgo biloba (Le Bars et al 1997) — CGIC
□ Placebo   ◇ Ginkgo biloba Egb
(No effect seen)

were of differing lengths and different instruments were used in each study, no direct comparison can be made between treatments.

Future developments in assessing symptoms

Global assessments bring a measure of real life into the assessment of anti-dementia drug efficacy. Within the assessment there is always the opportunity for the patient and caregiver to express their opinions. This subjectivity, combined with the blinded opinions of individual clinicians, makes a positive outcome on a global assessment a convincing proof of drug efficacy.

Future developments will probably focus on the structure and nature of the background assessment upon which the rating is based, and the anchor points or guidelines for the ratings themselves. There is, however, a significant risk that if the assessment and rating becomes too structured then the measure will no longer be truly global, but will take on a psychometric profile. In particular, early recommendations to anchor the seven-point change scale degrees of change in patient functional independence (Knopman et al 1994), have been criticized as turning the measure into another functional scale, discounting cognitive or behavioural change (Doody et al 1998).

Current anti-dementia drugs are of modest effect at best. Many of the issues of sensitivity and reliability in global ratings are a direct consequence of the problems of trying to measure very small changes. More effective drugs will have a more dramatic effect on global ratings. The inherent advantages of taking in the broadest picture means that global measures will undoubtedly remain mandatory outcome measures in clinical trials for the foreseeable future.

Acknowledgements

Richard Harvey is supported by an Alzheimer's Disease Society Research Fellowship.

References

Berg L (1988) Clinical dementia rating (CDR). *Psychopharmacol Bull* **24**:637–9.

Corey-Bloom J, Anand R, Veach J for the ENA 713 B352 Study Group (1998). A randomized trial evaluating the efficacy and safety of ENA 713 (rivastigmine tartrate), a new acetylcholinesterase inhibitor, in patients with mild to moderately severe Alzheimer's disease. *Int J Geriat Psychopharmacol* **1**:55–65.

Doody RS, Wimo A, Jonsson B et al (1998) In: Test scores in clinical trials vs performance in real life: can clinical global assessments bridge the gap? In: *Health Economics of Dementia*. John Wiley & Sons: Chichester, 311–25.

Guy W (1976) *ECDEU Assessment Manual for Psychopharmacology.* US Department of Health and Human Services: Rockville, MD: Clinical Global Impressions (CGI), 218–22.

Kewitz H, Berzewski H, Rainer M (1994) Galanthamine, a selective nontoxic avetyl-cholinesterase inhibitor is significantly superior over placebo in the treatment of SDAT [Abstract]. *Neuropsychopharmacology* **10**(Suppl 2):130.

Knopman DS, Knapp MJ, Gracon SI, Davis CS (1994) The Clinician Interview-Based Impression (CIBI) — a clinician global change rating-scale in Alzheimer's disease. *Neurol* **44**:2315–21.

Le Bars PL, Katz MM, Berman N et al and the North American EGb Study Group (1997). A placebo-controlled, double-blind, randomized trial of an extract of Ginkgo biloba for dementia. North American EGb Study Group. *JAMA* **278**:1327–32.

Leber P (1990) *Guidelines for the clinical evaluation of antidementia drugs.* US Food and Drug Administration: Rockville MD.

Marcusson J, Rother M, Kittner B et al (1997) A 12–month, randomized, placebo-controlled trial of propentofylline (HWA 285) in patients with dementia according to DSM III-R. The European Propentofylline Study Group. *Dement Geriatr Cogn Disord* **8**:320–8.

Reisberg B (1988) Functional assessment staging. *Psychopharmacol Bull* **24**:653–9.

Reisberg B, Ferris SH (1994) *CIBIC-Plus interview guide.* Sandoz Pharmaceuticals Corporation: East Hannover, NJ.

Reisberg B, Ferris SH, de Leon MJ, Crook T (1982) The global deterioration scale for assessment of primary degenerative dementia. *Am J Psychiatry* **139**:1136–9.

Rogers SL, Farlow MR, Mohs R, Friedhoff LT and the Donepezil Study Group (1998). A 24-week, double-blind, placebo-controlled trial of donepezil in patients with Alzheimer's disease. *Neurol* **50**:136–45.

Schneider LS, Olin JT (1997) Clinical global impressions in clinical trials. *Int Psychogeriatrics* **8**:277–90.

Schneider LS, Olin JT, Doody RS et al (1997) Validity and reliability of the Alzheimer's disease cooperative study-clinical global impression of change. *Alzheimer Dis Assoc Disord* **11**(Suppl 2):S22–S32.

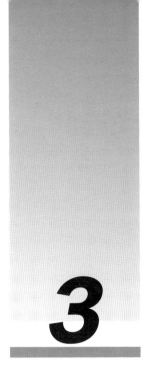

Activities of daily living

3

Introduction

Changes in function are so intrinsic to Alzheimer's disease that they are considered as independent criteria for the diagnosis (McKhann et al 1984). However, functional decline is in itself not a precise concept — which functions and in what contexts? Activities of daily living (ADLs) are an attempt to operationalize this increasing inability to function in daily life that comes with the dementia. Assessment measures for ADLs have been described that have acceptable reliability and validity. Each of the domains of decline in Alzheimer's disease invokes a specific treatment-need but of all these domains the loss of ADL ability is the main determinant of social and continuing care needs. It is the level of ADL ability that dictates the services required at home and, ultimately, it is the loss of ADL activity that determines the timing of entry into residential or continuing nursing care (Riter and Fries 1992). The importance of a thorough assessment of ADL abilities cannot therefore be overemphasized, and equally any change in ADL activity resulting from treatment will be a major advance with wide implications.

What are ADLs?

Activities of daily living can be grouped as those that relate to self-care and instrumental activities; both those relating to the immediate environment (home) and those relating to the wider environment (neighbourhood). Self-care ADLs are principally dressing and personal hygiene. Dressing abilities are lost gradually; initially difficulties arise with doing up cufflinks or jewellery, progressing to difficulties with buttons and buckles, through to items put on incorrectly or in the wrong order. In time the ability to dress is lost with carers needing first to prompt, then to assist in dressing and finally to take over the task completely. Personal hygiene follows the same course; initially make-up is not put on as well or hair is less groomed, then teeth are not brushed as well as dentures not cleaned, baths are taken less often and prompting is needed before finally the carer is required to assume the task of self-hygiene completely.

Instrumental ADLs related to the immediate environment include housework, cooking, and using household devices. The previously immaculate house will begin to acquire a veneer of dust, the previously accomplished cook will struggle using the oven and the washing machine will be used less often or incorrectly. As the disorder progresses housework, cooking or using the machines we are surrounded with becomes impossible.

As ADL abilities are lost often the patient will retreat into the home. Shopping, negotiating public transport and other ADLs related to the wider environment become increasingly difficult. Driving is a special case and needs particular attention. It goes without saying that driving requires considerable cognitive and manual skills and these are compromised early in the dementia process. Continuing to drive places the affected person and, of course, many others at considerable risk.

Change in ADLs in Alzheimer's disease

The decline in the domain of ADLs is the outward manifestation of the global decline of dementia, and in Alzheimer's disease it seems to follow a moderately predictable course. It has been claimed that not only is the course of loss of ADL ability similar between patients but there is a moderately high degree of concordance between loss of functional ability and decline in cognitive abilities. A number of studies have broadly confirmed the uniform natural history, showing that the sequence of losses is similar for most but not all ADLs (Stern et al 1990; Green et al 1993; Reisberg et al 1986). The concordance between cognitive abilities and functional abilities is less clear cut. Individual assessment measures assessing ability in functional as well as cognitive domains show similar scores between these domains in individual patients implying that when one declines so does the other (Rockwood and Morris 1996; Reisberg et al 1989). However, other studies have reported discordance between cognition and function (Teri et al 1989; Reed et al 1989). It would seem that functional ability is related to, but not entirely dependent upon, cognitive abilities — there are individual factors that relate to a particular person's functional capacity.

It may be that there are biological substrates to this individual variability in functional decline as there appear to be for variability in the behaviourial domain (Holmes et al 1996; Forstl et al 1994) but these remain to be determined. However, it is clear that other factors including cultural and gender do affect functional ability. Just as prior ability affects assessment of cognition, prior ability also affects assessment of function. Many elderly men, for example, have little prior cooking ability and so assessing function in the kitchen can be problematical. Within some communities the elderly live with younger members of the family and less function is expected than for the elderly living alone. Again assessing function can be misleading. In both of these cases assessment should be personalized and the change measured. The functional ability of an individual should be measured against what is normal and expected of them.

Assessment of ADL

Objectives

The assessment of ADL is critical to dementia care and to developing drug treatments although the objectives of assessment in each case differ. For the clinician determining functional ability is directed towards determining care needs. The introduction of home care, the transition to continuing or residential care is determined by the functional ability of the patient. Assessment should therefore be comprehensive enough to determine which activities of living were once accomplished but are now no longer and require intervention. For the researcher conducting a trial, assessment objectives are somewhat different in that assessment should be reliable between assessments and between researchers and sensitive to change.

Tools

Assessment of function, for both instrumental and basic ADL, can be by direct observation or by interview with the caregiver; both have a place, although in clinical trials the latter dominates.

Research instruments using direct observation with acceptable reliability and validity with respect to other instruments have been developed such as the Activities of Daily Living Situational Test (Skurla et al 1988) or the Direct Assessment of Function status. However, these are time-consuming assessments and in clinical trials assessments by caregiver interview such as the Progressive

Deterioration Scale (PDS; DeJong et al 1989) or the Interview for Deterioration in Daily Functioning Activities are used. Based upon a checklist of functions together with an assessment of severity either on an analogue scale or on a likert scale these assessments are reliable and valid and claim to be effective measures of change. However, like all scales in dementia assessment, floor and ceiling effects remain, linearity cannot be assumed (although usually is) and sensitivity to change remains to be established. Furthermore as discussed above, functional abilities, possibly more than the other domains, are highly influenced by gender, culture and, one suspects, cohort effects.

Such assessment procedures find little use in ordinary clinical practice — the cost-benefit in terms of time spent and information gained is poor. Simplified scales have been developed, however, that are ideal for routine clinical use and provide an important supplement to routine assessment. The Bristol Activities of Daily Living Scale is a short (20-item) scale covering both instrumental and self-care items that can be used as part of a structured interview or as a self-report questionnaire by carers (Bucks et al 1996). As such it is an excellent, uncomplicated addition to the clinical interview. The Functional Assessment Staging (FAST) scale developed by Reisberg is not an assessment tool but a description of the severity of Alzheimer's disease according to, in the simplest form, a seven-stage scale (Reisberg 1988). The FAST scale depends heavily upon the notion that deterioration in Alzheimer's disease is relatively uniform and in most cases follows a particular sequence. The FAST, like the Bristol ADL scale, has the merit of ease of use in addition to providing clinically-relevant information making it an ideal tool for routine clinical use.

These scales, and other similar ones, can be used by many members of the multidisciplinary team. However, interviews with caregivers and the use of ADL and functional scales provide only a guide to ability and the occupational therapist has a particularly important role in the assessment of functional impairment in addition to integrating assessment with treatment (Corcoran and Gitlin 1992). The occupational therapist's assessment will include a detailed and practical hands-on assessment of abilities with dressing and in the kitchen, and these will often be performed in the patient's own home.

The occupational therapist might assess shopping abilities by accompanying the person noting in the process the ability to remember short lists, topographical orientation, ability to handle money and, most importantly, safety on roads. The urban environment is hostile to elderly people at the best of times.

Driving is such an important activity of daily living and the consequences of failing function are so potentially disastrous that its importance cannot be over-emphasized. Dementia is almost certainly a contributing factor in a significant number of accidents (Carr 1997) and many drivers continue to drive after Alzheimer's disease has been diagnosed and functional ability is lost (Fox et al 1997). Screening tests for driving ability that can be used by the primary-care physician or specialist have been developed (Carr et al 1998) but there is probably no substitute for specialized on-road assessment of driving ability (Fox et al 1997; Fitten 1997). In the UK driving assessment centres will provide such an examination; further details can be obtained from the DVLA.

Managing functional decline

Functional decline in Alzheimer's disease can be managed and now with the arrival of therapies it is possible that functional decline can be treated. However, the prospect of treatment is unlikely to eclipse the reality of effective and clinically important management for some time to come. The first step in effective management is complete assessment which will include some combination of multidisciplinary assessment, caregivers' interviews and the use of reliable and validated scales.

The aim of assessment should be both to stage the functional decline and to highlight those particular functional areas that are causing most concern. Concerns might be focused on the patient, the carer and on others. Particular concern will be paid to safety although as function declines there is always a balance between tolerating risk and preserving autonomy. One of the most important advances in dementia care has been, in effect, to embrace the concept that although the person with functional impairments is vulnerable when living in the community this is tolerated in exchange for preserving quality of life by remaining in a familiar environment for as long as possible.

Management of functional impairments of those living in the community ranges from relatively minor household adjustments to provision of aids to providing domicilliary care. The role of the carer is vital, as it is with all aspects of dementia treatment. Despite the range of assistance to compensate for functional losses that can be provided, it is inevitably the carer that provides most. Carers should be involved in the assessment and provision of care and there are important differences between spouse and adult–child carers and between husband and wife carers for example (Corcoran 1992). Recognizing the importance of carers can delay entry into continuing care (Mittleman et al 1993).

The costs of Alzheimer's disease are very large indeed and a large part of these costs are incurred through continuing care. Reducing the length of stay in continuing care would result in a disproportionate reduction in costs and is a major aim in treatment programmes for Alzheimer's disease. In clinical practice it is functional ability that is the most important factor in deciding when an individual moves from community care to continuing care and a number of studies confirm that it is function that best predicts institutionalization (Scott et al 1997;

Severson 1994; Heyman 1997). Difficulties with ADL not only predict institutionalization but also mortality — probably reflecting the close correlation between function and other markers of severity (Bianchetti et al 1995)

Treating functional decline

It is not surprising that considerable efforts have been made to establish whether treatments for Alzheimer's disease, designed to rectify cognitive impairment, also effect function. ADLs have also been used as an outcome measure in trials of many different classes of compound (Sano et al 1997; Marcusson et al 1997; Oakley and Sunderland 1997; Maltby et al 1994). Of these, it is the acetylcholinesterase inhibitors that are approved for use in Alzheimer's disease and trials of donepezil, tacrine, rivastigmine and metrifonate have all demonstrated some effect on function as well as on cognition.

As an example, nearly 700 patients were randomized to placebo or to high or low dose rivastigmine (Corey-Bloom et al 1998). Those on placebo declined, by an average of nearly 5 points on the 29-point PDS as did those on the low dose drug. Those treated with the high dose, on the other hand, declined by an average of 1.5 (intention to treat analysis) with differences between treated and placebo at 18 and 26 weeks. Given the relative coarseness of the measures of function and the similarity in pharmacological action of the various compounds it is not surprising that similar effects for the other available acetylcholinesterase inhibitors have been reported.

Evaluating the relevance of such treatment effects, however, has been controversial. On the one hand, only modest differences between drug and placebo has led some to be sceptical as to the clinical relevance of such a difference. On the other hand the trials so far are all relatively short term and the treatment effect size is comparable to the decline over the course of the trial. As for the other domains, the acetylcholinesterase inhibitors appear to slow or even halt the decline in functional deterioration over the period measured. The effects of these compounds on long-term function remains to be seen.

Conclusions

Functional ability and ADL represent the outward face of the global decline that occurs in Alzheimer's disease. Functional loss accompanies cognitive loss but it is function, more than any other domain, that dictates the care needs of people with dementia and, ultimately dictates the need for continuing care. Functional losses can be managed although to do so well requires detailed assessment and appropriate provision of services. Assessment is a task for the multidisciplinary team with the occupational therapist having a special role, and at best, assessment is a combination of direct observation, interview with the caregiver and the use of validated scales. Improvement in the management of functional losses is one of the greatest challenges for Alzheimer's disease therapies and yet equally brings with it the greatest potential rewards.

References

Bianchetti A, Scuratti A, Zanetti O et al (1995) Predictors of mortality and institutionalization in Alzheimer disease patients 1 year after discharge from an Alzheimer dementia unit. *Dementia* **6**:108–12.

Bucks RS, Ashworth DL, Wilcock GK, Siegfried K (1996) Assessment of activities of daily living in dementia: development of the Bristol Activities of Daily Living Scale. *Age Ageing* **25**:113–20.

Carr DB (1997) Motor vehicle crashes and drivers with DAT. *Alzheimer Dis Assoc Disord* **11**(Suppl 1):38–41.

Carr DB, LaBarge E, Dunnigan K, Storandt M (1998) Differentiating drivers with dementia of the Alzheimer type from healthy older persons with a traffic sign naming test. *J Gerontol [A]* **53A**:M135–M139.

Corcoran MA (1992) Gender differences in dementia management plans of spousal caregivers: implications for occupational therapy. *Am J Occup Ther* **46**:1006–12.

Corcoran MA, Gitlin LN (1992) Dementia management: an occupational therapy home-based intervention for caregivers. *Am J Occup Ther* **46**:801–8.

Corey-Bloom J, Anand J, Veach J (1998) A randomized trial evaluating the efficacy and safety of ENA 713 (rivastigmine tartrate), a new acetylcholinesterase inhibitor, in patients with mild to moderately severe Alzheimer's disease. *Int J Geriat Psychopharmacol* **1**:55–65.

DeJong R, Osterlund OW, Roy GW (1989) Measurement of quality-of-life changes in patients with Alzheimer's disease. *Clin Ther* **11**:545–54.

Fitten LJ (1997) The demented driver: The doctor's dilemma. *Alzheimer Dis Assoc Disord* **11**(Suppl 1):57–61.

Forstl H, Burns A, Levy R, Cairns N (1994) Neuropathological correlates of psychotic phenomena in confirmed Alzheimer's disease. *Br J Psychiatry* **165**:53–9.

Fox GK, Bowden SC, Bashford GM, Smith DS (1997) Alzheimer's disease and driving: Prediction and assessment of driving performance. *J Am Geriatr Soc* **45**:949–53.

Green CR, Mohs RC, Schmeidler et al (1993) Functional decline in Alzheimer's disease: a longitudinal study. *J Am Geriatr Soc* **41**:654–61.

Heyman A, Peterson B, Fillenbaum G, Pieper C (1997) Predictors of time to institutionalization of patients with Alzheimer's disease: The CERAD experience. *Neurology* **48**:1304–9.

Holmes C, Levy R, McLoughlin DM et al (1996) Apolipoprotein E and the clinical features of late onset Alzheimer's disease. *J Neurol Neurosurg Psychiatry* **61**:580–3.

McKhann G, Drachman D, Folstein M et al (1984) Clinical diagnosis of Alzheimer's disease: report of the NINCDS-ADRDA Work Group under the auspices of Department of Health and Human Services Task Force on Alzheimer's Disease. *Neurology* **34**:939–44.

Marcusson J, Rother M, Kittner B et al (1997) A 12-month, randomized, placebo-controlled trial of propentofylline (HWA 285) in patients with dementia according to DSM III-R. *Dementia* **8**:320–8.

Maltby N, Broe GA, Greasey H et al (1994) Efficacy of tacrine and lecithin in mild to moderate Alzheimer's disease: double blind trial. *BMJ* **308**:879–83.

Mittelman MS, Ferris SH, Steinberg G, Shulman E (1993) An intervention that delays institutionalization of Alzheimer's disease patients: Treatment of spouse-caregivers. *Gerontologist* **33**:730–40.

Oakley F, Sunderland T (1997) Assessment of motor and process skills as a measure of IADL functioning in pharmacologic studies of people with Alzheimer's disease: a pilot study. *Int Psychogeriatr* **9**:197–206.

Reed BR, Jagust WJ, Seab JP (1989) Mental status as a predictor of daily function in progressive dementia. *Gerontologist* **29**:804–7.

Reisberg B (1988) Functional assessment staging (FAST). *Psychopharmacol Bull* **24**:653–9.

Reisberg B, Ferris SH, Shulman E et al (1986) Longitudinal course of normal aging and progressive dementia of the Alzheimer's type: a prospective study of 106 subjects over a 3.6 year mean interval. *Prog Neuropsychopharmacol Biol Psychiatry* **10**:571–8.

Reisberg B, Ferris SH, De Leon MJ et al (1989) The stage specific temporal course of Alzheimer's disease: functional and behavioral concomitants based upon cross-sectional and longitudinal observation. *Prog Clin Biol Res* **317**:23–41.

Riter RN, Fries BE (1992) Predictors of the placement of cognitively impaired residents on special care units. *Gerontologist* **32**:184–90.

Rockwood K, Morris JC (1996) Global staging methods in dementia. In: Gauthier S (ed) *Clinical Diagnosis and Management of Alzheimer's Disease*. Martin Dunitz, London: 141–53.

Sano M, Ernesto C, Thomas RG et al (1997) A controlled trial of selegiline, alpha-tocopherol, or both as treatment for Alzheimer's disease. *N Engl J Med* **336**:1216–22.

Scott WK, Edwards KB, Davis DR et al (1997) Risk of institutionalization among community long-term care clients with dementia. *Gerontologist* **37**:46–51.

Severson MA, Smith GE, Tangalos EG et al (1994) Patterns and predictors of institutionalization in community-based dementia patients. *J Am Geriatr Soc* **42**:181–5.

Skurla E, Rogers JC, Sunderland T (1988) Direct assessment of activities of daily living in Alzheimer's disease. A controlled study. *J Am Geriatr Soc* **36**:97–103.

Stern Y, Hesdorffer D, Sano M, Mayeux R (1990) Measurement and prediction of functional capacity in Alzheimer's disease. *Neurology* **40**:8–14.

Teri L, Borson S, Kiyak HA, Yamagishi M (1989) Behavioral disturbance, cognitive dysfunction, and functional skill. Prevalence and relationship in Alzheimer's disease. *J Am Geriatr Soc* **37**:109–16.

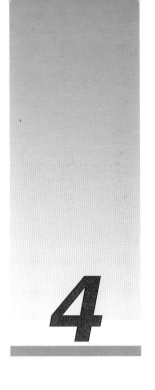

Neuropsychiatric symptoms

Objectives of assessment

Assessment of neuropsychiatric symptoms and behavioural changes in patients with Alzheimer's disease (AD) is a critical part of a comprehensive evaluation and is imperative for quality care. Neuropsychiatric symptoms are common in AD and are responsible for a substantial amount of the morbidity associated with the disease. Psychiatric symptoms such as paranoia, anxiety and depression produce marked patient distress. Furthermore, agitation, delusions, irritability, lability and mood changes are important sources of distress for the carer. Behavioural changes are one of the principal reasons that carers decide to institutionalize patients, and patients in extended care facilities have greater frequencies and severities of behavioural disturbances than community-dwelling patients. Neuropsychiatric symptoms, such as paranoia or anxiety, may precipitate aggression by the patient or abuse by the carer. Most investigations have found that behavioural disturbances are a greater source of carer distress than the memory abnormalities and cognitive decline of AD. Many of the neuropsychiatric symptoms of AD are treatable with cholinergic agents or psychotropic drugs, and amelioration of these symptoms has benefit both for patients and carers. Reduction in behavioural disturbances may also defer nursing home placement and reduce costs associated with institutional care. Thus, assessment of the neuropsychiatric domain of AD is important in understanding the patient, providing insight into carer burden, and informing non-pharmacologic and pharmacologic intervention.

Symptoms to be assessed

Alzheimer's disease produces a wide array of neuropsychiatric symptoms (**Figure 4.1**; Mega et al 1996). Apathy is the most common behavioural change evidenced by patients with AD. Early in the clinical course, in concert with the onset of memory abnormalities, patients manifest progressive emotional distancing, loss of interest, disengagement, reduced motivation, and decreased initiation. These symptoms are disproportionate to the accompanying cognitive impairment

and may not be accompanied by reduced physical activity. Apathy is present in approximately half of the patients in the early phases of the illness and is evident in nearly all of them in the final stages of AD.

Agitation is also common in AD. It becomes progressively more frequent as the disease progresses, and brief periods of agitation may be present early in the disease. Agitation is a non-specific behavioural syndrome which includes shouting, cursing, hitting, shoving, and actively resisting the provision of care. In some cases agitation is a response to pain, urinary retention, faecal impaction, infection or fever; in others, it is a response to overstimulation, excessive noise, or restraint. Anxiety, delusions and hallucinations may also lead to agitation. In some cases no accompanying potentially causal issues can be discovered. In all patients, a search for remedial and environmental circumstances must be pursued before treatment of agitation with pharmacological agents is initiated.

Mood changes are also common in AD. Depressive symptoms may occasionally precede the onset of cognitive abnormalities, and depression-scale scores

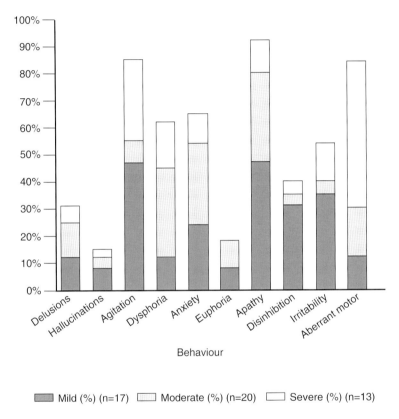

Figure 4.1
Percent of patients in different stages of Alzheimer's disease manifesting behavioural changes as measured by the Neuropsychiatric Inventory (Mega et al 1998).

tend to increase as the disease progresses. It is unusual for patients with AD and depression to meet all of the criteria of the fourth edition of the Diagnostic and Statistical Manual of Mental Disorders (DSM-IV) (American Psychiatric Association 1994) for Major Depressive Episode, but dysphoria, dysthymia, and minor depressive syndromes are common. Alzheimer's disease unaccompanied by mood changes can produce apathy, weight loss, agitation and sleep disturbances; identification of a depression syndrome in AD depends on recognition of core psychological features including sadness, feelings of worthlessness and helplessness, convictions of hopelessness, and thoughts of death.

Personality alterations are a frequent occurrence in AD. Approximately half of the patients will exhibit irritability and emotional lability, and approximately one-third will have increased tactlessness and impulsiveness and reduced empathy.

Anxiety is a common manifestation of AD, occurring in half of the patients. Patients may become anxious in novel circumstances, and in some cases cannot tolerate being separated from their carer for even short periods of time.

Finally, there are a wide range of other behavioural disturbances that do not fit conveniently into traditional psychiatric classifications. These include purposeless motor activity such as pacing, rummaging in drawers and closets, and wandering. Misidentification syndromes such as mirror sign (ie, when the patient does not recognize themselves in the mirror and is convinced that someone is watching them) or picture

sign (ie, where the patient believes that individuals on television are actually present in the home) may be manifestations of the cognitive disturbance of AD or part of a psychotic disorder. In addition, some patients may have sexually inappropriate or aggressive behaviours.

Approaches to the assessment of neuropsychiatric symptoms

Syndromic diagnoses

The neuropsychiatric manifestations of AD may be approached as syndromes, symptoms, or a combination of both. The DSM-IV (American Psychiatric Association 1994) and the Tenth Revision of the International Classification of Diseases (ICD-10) (World Health Organization 1992) employ the syndromic approach to neuropsychiatric diagnosis. Using DSM-IV, patients with neuropsychiatric symptoms would be identified as suffering from AD and would be specified further as AD with delusions, AD with depressed mood, or AD with behavioural disturbance, depending on the accompanying behavioural manifestations. ICD-10 uses a dual syndrome approach—patients with AD and depression would simultaneously meet syndromic criteria for AD and separate syndromic criteria for depression, psychosis or other behavioural symptoms. Information for these syndromic diagnoses are typically derived from a combination of carer report and clinician observation of the patient. Criteria are not fully operationalized and severity or frequency ratings are not incorporated. The elements of the syndromes can be converted into a checklist, and structured interviews for the syndromes have been developed. These structured interviews tend to be time- and labour-intensive and do not lend themselves to non-research clinical settings, but are excellent research tools.

Rating scales

Rating scales may identify syndromes, symptoms, or a mixture. The Neuropsychiatric Inventory (Cummings et al 1994), developed to assess psychopathology in dementia patients, groups individual symptoms into complexes. For example, delusions of theft and infidelity comprise part of the delusion symptom complex. Similar symptom groupings are used to identify symptom complexes corresponding to hallucinations, agitation, dysphoria, anxiety, euphoria, apathy, disinhibition, irritability, and aberrant or purposeless

motor activity. Each symptom is rated by the caregiver for its frequency and severity. The BEHAVE-AD (Reisberg et al 1987) uses a similar approach, identifying symptom complexes including paranoid and delusional ideation, hallucinations, activity disturbances, aggressiveness, diurnal rhythm disturbances, affective disturbances, and anxieties and phobias. Each item of the symptom complexes is scored for its severity. The Behavioral Rating Scale for Dementia (Tariot et al 1995) used factor analysis to group 51 symptoms into eight factors including depressive features, psychotic features, defective self-regulation, irritability/agitation, vegetative features, apathy, aggression, and affective lability. Each of the 51 items is rated for frequency based on the caregiver's report. Some scales include the caregiver's reactions to neuropsychiatric symptoms. For example, the Neuropsychiatric Inventory assesses the degree of carer distress produced by each behavioural disturbance (Kaufer et al 1998a).

Some instruments widely used in dementia research concentrate on specific types of behavioural abnormalities. The Cohen-Mansfield Agitation Inventory (Koss et al 1997) provides a detailed assessment of agitation applicable primarily to patients in residential settings. The Cornell Scale for Depression in Dementia (Alexopoulos 1988) focuses on the identification of depressive syndromes in patients with AD and other dementias.

A variety of other tools have been developed for use in specific circumstances or to answer research and clinical questions. In the clinical setting, the most common items from these instruments can be used as simple checklists to alert the clinician to the presence of behavioural disturbances.

The use of standardized rating scales has advanced the understanding of the neuropsychiatric domain of AD. Operationalized criteria, scripted questions and defined anchor points for ratings all serve to improve the reliability of data collected and reduce dependence on clinician expertise. To be implemented with confidence, rating scales should be shown to have acceptable inter-rater reliability (ie, when the scale is administered by two different clinicians, similar scores are achieved), test–retest reliability (ie, when the test is given twice in a short interval of time, the carer provides similar responses), and concurrent

validity (ie, the instrument provides information similar to that obtained by a 'gold standard' existing instrument). Multidimensional instruments such as the Neuropsychiatric Inventory, BEHAVE-AD and Behavioral Rating Scale for Dementia assess many neuropsychiatric domains in AD but provide less information on specific domains than syndromic-specific scales such as the Cohen-Mansfield Agitation Inventory or the Cornell Scale for Depression in Dementia. Some scales require more time and depend on asking every question, whereas others such as the Neuropsychiatric Inventory use a screening methodology to save administration time.

Current therapies of neuropsychiatric symptoms

General principles

Cholinergic therapies of AD ameliorate a variety of the neuropsychiatric manifestations. In addition, treatment with antidepressants, conventional and novel antipsychotics, anxiolytics, anti-agitation agents, and sedative-hypnotics reduce specific behavioural disturbances (Wright and Cummings 1996; see **Table 4.1**). Pharmacological conservatism is in order when considering treatment of

Table 4.1
Drugs commonly used to treat behavioural disturbances in Alzheimer's disease (Wright and Cummings 1996).

Treatment	Daily oral dose range (mg)	Treatment	Daily oral dose range (mg)
Agitation and aggression		**Anxiety**	
Mood stabilizing agents		Lorazepam	0.5–4
Carbamazepine	100–1000	Oxazepam	10–30
Divalproex	250–3000	Propranolol	10–160
Antidepressants		Buspirone	15–45
Trazodone	150–500	**Depression**	
Anxiolytics		Selective serotonin reuptake inhibitors	
Buspirone	15–45	Citalopram	10–40
Lorazepam	0.5–6	Fluoxetine	20–80
Beta-blockers		Paroxetine	10–40
Propranolol	60–520	Sertraline	50–200
Antipsychotics		Fluvoxamine	50–300
Haloperidol	0.5–3		
Risperidone	0.5–2.0	Tricyclic antidepressants	
Olanzapine	5–15	Desipramine	50–150
Quetiapine	25–250	Nortriptyline	50–100
		Other antidepressants	
Psychosis		Nefazodone	300–600
Antipsychotics		Venlafaxine	75–375
Haloperidol	0.5–3	**Insomnia**	
Risperidone	0.5–2.0	Trazodone	50–300
Olanzapine	5–15	Zolpidem	5–10
Quetiapine	25–250	Temazepam	15–30

neuropsychiatric symptoms in AD. Non-pharmacological interventions should be implemented prior to initiating drug therapy.

One approach to non-pharmacological intervention utilizes an 'A-B-C' approach. 'A' stands for the antecedents of behaviour and indicates the need to analyse the circumstances that may have contributed to precipitating a behavioural event. 'B' stands for the behaviour itself and requires considera-tion of the meaning of the behaviour

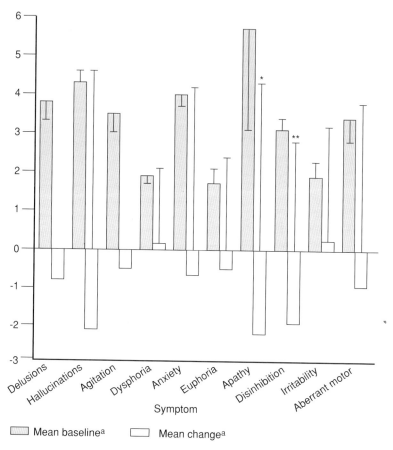

Figure 4.2
Neuropsychiatric Inventory scores before and after treatment with tacrine.
[a]Mean (±SD) NPI baseline and change scores include those with emergent symptoms
*Wilcoxon signed-rank test, P = 0.011
**Wilcoxon signed-rank test, P = 0.05

from the patient and carer perspective. 'C' stands for the consequences of the behaviour and indicates the need to consider what follows as a behavioural event to ensure that behavioural disturbances are not being reinforced by attention from the carer or some other positive reward. In addition, attention to the needs of the carer with referral to the Alzheimer's Association and identification of community resources may help to decrease the burden of the carer, allowing them to respond to behavioural disturbances in more positive ways. These interventions may make it possible to avoid drug treatment.

In some cases, pharmacological treatment cannot be avoided. Medications should be started in low doses and increased only after symptom response at the previous dose has been assessed. Doses should be increased to maximal benefit or emergence of side effects. Neuropsychiatric symptoms fluctuate over time and some disappear spontaneously during the course of the illness. Thus, reassessment of the need for psychotropic medication should be made at each clinic visit. Compliance, side effects, and drug interactions are other aspects of pharmacotherapy with which the clinician should be familiar.

Cholinesterase inhibitor therapy

Cholinesterase inhibitors are used primarily for cognitive enhancement in AD. However, the cholinergic disturbance of AD makes an important contribution to the behavioural manifestations, and reduction of the cholinergic deficiency may have beneficial behavioural effects (Cummings and Kaufer 1996). Tacrine has been shown to reduce apathy, anxiety, disinhibition and aberrant/purposeless motor behaviour (Kaufer et al 1998b; **Figure 4.2**) and metrifonate to reduce the total score on the Neuropsychiatric Inventory as well as visual hallucinations (Morris et al 1998; **Figure 4.3**). Preliminary investigation of other cholinesterase inhibitors suggests that behavioural improvement may be a class-related property of these agents associated with their cholinergic-enhancing properties. Tacrine donepezil, metrifonate, rivastigmine, galantamine, long-acting physostigmine, and eptastigmine are cholinesterase inhibitors that are available or are under study. Total scores on behavioural rating instruments as well as item scores on apathy and visual hallucinations tend to respond best to cholinomimetic therapy. Agitation, delusions, anxiety, disinhibition, depression and aberrant motor behaviour have shown a beneficial response to cholinergic therapy in some studies.

Antipsychotic agents

Antipsychotic agents reduce delusions, hallucinations and agitation in patients

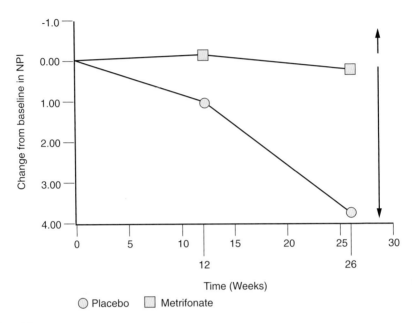

Figure 4.3
Total Neuropsychiatric Inventory score over 24 weeks of treatment with metrifonate. There is significant behavioural deterioration in the group on placebo compared to the metrifonate-treated group.

with AD manifesting these symptoms. Double-blind, placebo-controlled studies have been rare and, where available, suggest that the magnitude of the response is modest. Conventional neuroleptics such as haloperidol are commonly used. They may produce adverse extrapyramidal symptoms, and monitoring for parkinsonism and tardive dyskinesia is mandatory. Novel antipsychotics, including risperidone, olanzapine and quetiapine, reduce psychosis in AD and cause fewer extrapyramidal reactions.

Antidepressants

The depression syndrome of AD exacerbates disability and produces distress in both patient and caregiver. Amelioration of the mood disturbance can be pursued with traditional antidepressants. Selective serotonin reuptake inhibitors have fewer side effects than tricyclic agents and comprise the drugs of choice in this situation. Citalopram, sertraline, fluoxetine, paroxetine or fluvoxamine may be used. If patients fail to respond to a selective serotonin reuptake inhibitor, then treatment with a tricyclic agent with few anticholinergic side effects may be attempted. Nortriptyline or desipramine may be used. Agents that have combined actions on serotonin and noradrenaline, such as venlafaxine, may have a role in the management of apathetic and depressive syndromes in AD.

Anti-agitation agents

Psychotic patients with agitation should be treated with antipsychotic agents as described above. Patients with agitation occurring primarily during the night may be improved with treatment with sedative-hypnotics including trazodone, zolpidem or Temazepam. Mood stabilizing drugs are increasingly used to reduce daytime agitation in patients with AD. Divalproex or carbamazepine reduce agitation and have fewer side effects than many psychotropic agents.

Anxiolytics

Benzodiazepines are generally avoided in AD because they may increase confusion or exacerbate disinhibition. Patients with infrequent episodes of agitation may respond to single doses of a benzodiazepine such as lorazepam or oxazepam. These drugs are well metabolized in the elderly and have less tendency to accumulate over time. For patients requiring daily anxiolytic therapy, treatment with buspirone may be a superior alternative. In some cases, treatment with propranolol may be beneficial.

Sedative-hypnotics

Sleep abnormalities are common in AD and disturb both patient and carer. Sedative-hypnotics that may aid in sleep induction and provide sleep maintenance for at least a few hours include trazodone, zolpidem and temazepam. Long-acting benzodiazepines and barbiturates should be avoided.

Disease-modifying therapies

Antioxidant therapies such as vitamin E and selegiline, and anti-inflammatory agents such as nonsteroidal anti-inflammatory drugs (NSAIDs) may defer the

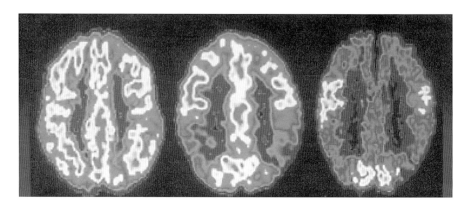

Figure 4.4
Fluorodeoxyglucose positron emission tomogram of a normal elderly individual (left), a patient with Alzheimer's disease without behavioural disturbances (centre), and a patient with Alzheimer's disease complicated by psychosis and disinhibition (right).

onset or slow the progression of AD. These agents have limited or no effect on existing symptoms of AD but may retard the emergence of new symptoms by slowing the progression of the disease. Most behavioural disturbances become more common over the course of AD, and slowing the progression of the illness would have the effect of moderating the emergence of new behavioural symptoms. Existing symptoms must be treated with cholinesterase inhibitors or psychotropic drugs as described above. A typical regimen for an AD patient will probably include several agents. Initiation of disease-modifying therapy with vitamin E and a

cholinesterase inhibitor should be followed by a period of observation to determine if behavioural disturbances are reduced. If intolerable neuropsychiatric symptoms persist after introduction of these agents, then a psychotropic drug should be added to this regimen.

Future developments in assessment and treatment

Alzheimer's disease patients with behavioural disturbances are biologically distinct from those without. Greater frontal lobe hypometabolism on fluorodeoxyglucose positron emission tomography has been found in patients with agitation, psychosis, apathy or depression, compared to patients without these symptoms (**Figure 4.4**; Hirono et al 1998; Sultzer et al 1995).

Preliminary neurobiological investigations suggest differences in the density of neuritic plaques and distribution of neurofibrillary tangles as well as neurochemical distinctions between patients with AD and psychosis compared to those with AD and no accompanying psychosis. Additional studies are necessary to determine the neurobiological correlates of behavioural disturbances in AD as a means to optimize mechanism-based therapy of these important disease manifestations.

Current studies of the psychotropic effects of cholinergic agents have been based primarily on studies of patients selected for the degree of cognitive disturbance rather than their specific behavioural symptoms. Clinical trials of patients selected for specific behavioural abnormalities are required for a comprehensive assessment of the psychotropic properties of these agents. In addition, many patients will be treated with combinations of anticholinesterase inhibitors plus other psychotropic agents including anti-psychotics, antidepressants, anti-epileptic agents, anxiolytics or sedative-hypnotics, and the effects of these drug combinations require investigation.

Combinations of cholinesterase inhibitors, antioxidants, (vitamin E, selegiline), hormonal therapies (oestrogen replacement), NSAIDS, and psychotropic agents can also be anticipated and warrant study.

Acknowledgements

This project was supported by a National Institute of Aging Alzheimer's Disease Center grant (AG 10123), an Alzheimer's Disease Research Center of California grant, and the Sidell-Kagan Foundation.

References

Alexopoulos GS, Abrams RC, Young RC, Shamoian CA (1988) Cornell Scale for Depression in Dementia. *Biol Psychiat* **23**:271–84.

American Psychiatric Association (1994) *Diagnostic and Statistical Manual of Mental Disorders, 4th edn.* American Psychiatric Association, Washington, DC.

Cummings JL, Kaufer D (1996) Neuropsychiatric aspects of Alzheimer's disease: The cholinergic hypothesis revisited. *Neurology* **47**:876–83.

Cummings JL, Mega M, Gray K et al (1994) The Neuropsychiatric Inventory: comprehensive assessment of psychopathology in dementia. *Neurology* **44**:2308–14.

Hirono N, Mori E, Ishii K et al (1998) Frontal lobe hypometabolism and depression in Alzheimer's disease. *Neurology* **50**:380–3.

Kaufer DI, Cummings JL, Christine D et al (1998a) Assessing the impact of neuropsychiatric symptoms in Alzheimer's disease: The Neuropsychiatric Inventory Caregiver Distress Scale. *J Am Geriatr Soc* **46**:210–5.

Kaufer D, Cummings JL, Christine D (1998b) Differential neuropsychiatric symptom responses to tacrine in Alzheimer's disease: Relationship to dementia severity. *J Neuropsychiatr Clin Neurosci* **10**:55–63.

Koss E, Weiner M, Ernesto C et al and the Alzheimer's Disease Cooperative Study (1997) Assessing patterns of agitation in Alzheimer's disease patients with the Cohen-Mansfield Agitation Inventory. *Alzheimer Dis Assoc Disord* **11**(Suppl 2):S4–S50.

Mega MS, Cummings JL, Fiorello T, Gornbein J (1996) The spectrum of behavioural changes in Alzheimer's disease. *Neurology* **46**:130–5.

Morris JC, Cyrus PA, Orazem J et al (1998) Metrifonate benefits cognitive, behavioural, and global function in patients with Alzheimer's disease. *Neurology* **50**:1222–30.

Reisberg B, Borenstein J, Salob SP et al (1987) Behavioral symptoms in Alzheimer's disease: Phenomenology and treatment. *J Clin Psychiatr* **48**(Suppl 5):9–15.

Sultzer DL, Mahler ME, Mandelkern MA et al (1995) The relationship between psychiatric symptoms and regional cortical metabolism in Alzheimer's disease. *J Neuropsychiatr Clin Neurosci* **7**:476–84.

Tariot PN, Mack JL, Patterson MB et al and the Behavioral Pathology Committee of the consortium to Establish a Registry for Alzheimer's Disease (1995) The Behavior Rating Scale for Dementia of the Consortium to Establish a Registry for Alzheimer's Disease. *Am J Psychiatr* **152**:1349–57.

World Health Organization (1992) *The ICD-10 Classification of Mental and Behavioural Disorders*. World Health Organization: Geneva, Switzerland.

Wright MT, Cummings JL (1996) Neuropsychiatric disturbances in Alzheimer's disease and other dementias: Recognition and management. *The Neurologist* **2**:207–18.

Quality of life

5

Objectives of assessment

The World Health Organization has defined quality of life (QOL) as:

> *'The individual's perceptions of their position in life in the context of the culture and value system in which they live, and in relationship to their goals, expectations, standards and concerns'*

This is clearly a complex and wide-reaching definition and so, in the clinical setting, it is more common to define QOL operationally as a multidimensional construct comprising physical, psychological and social well-being.

Quality of life measures have been developed for a number of reasons (**Table 5.1**; Fitzpatrick et al 1992) and are an established outcome in many therapeutic areas. More recently, attention has turned to the

Table 5.1
Applications of quality of life measures.

Screening and monitoring for psychosocial problems in individual patient care
Population surveys of perceived health problems
Medical audit
Outcome measures in health services or evaluation research
Clinical trials
Cost-utility analyses
(From Fitzpatrick et al 1992)

Table 5.2
QOL in dementia: proposed definitional models.

Lawton 1994	Psychological well-being; perceived QOL; behavioural competence; objective environment
Jones et al 1986	Survival safety/security; purpose; independence (based on Maslow's hierarchy of needs). (Theoretical underpinning of instrument development)
Brod and Stewart 1994	Physical functioning; daily activities (recreational, instrumental, work); mobility; social functioning and well-being; bodily well-being; positive and negative affective states; sense of aesthetics; self-concept and overall life satisfaction. (Framework built on literature review plus focus groups as first step to instrument development)
DeLetter et al 1995	Social interaction; basic physical care; appearance of patient to others and nutrition. (Factor analysis at stage of instrument development)

assessment of QOL in patients with dementia and such data are becoming increasingly important for a number of reasons. For example, despite the licensing of two new anti-dementia drugs in the UK (Kelly et al 1997), uptake of treatment has been limited, at least in part, by the lack of evidence of the effect on the sufferer's QOL. Moreover, the cost-effectiveness of available treatments and care is now under scrutiny, and many pharmacoeconomic studies include a QOL component, which is increasingly viewed as an important outcome (Revichi 1996). At present, QOL data in dementia, concerning either outcome of treatment of economic analyses, is scant.

Symptoms assessed

The three component model of QOL, comprising physical, psychological and social well-being, which are subjectively assessed, is the most common basis of QOL measurement in other therapeutic areas. This model, however, probably needs to be revised for dementia (Lawton 1994; Jones et al 1986; Brod and Stewart 1994; DeLetter et al 1995), and a number of alternative models have been proposed (**Table 5.2**) based upon areas thought to define QOL for the sufferer.

Assessment of QOL in any patient is complex, and the process is even more difficult in the patient with a degenerating, dementing condition. Methodological complexities (Whitehouse et al 1997; Lawton 1997; Stewart et al 1996) in this patient group arise for a number of reasons:

> - *Decreasing cognitive ability, limiting the patient's ability to introspect*
> - *Impaired communication skills*
> - *Discrepancies between subjective views (patient self-report) and objective views (caregiver or other proxy)*
> - *Anosognosia (the patient may be unaware of their deficits) or denial*

> *(the patient may not acknowledge their decreasing abilities)*
> - *The need to assess neuropsychiatric symptoms and behavioural problems in addition to cognitive impairment*
> - *Large differences in abilities at each stage of dementia*

Tools used

General measurement issues

Any new measuring instrument must undergo rigorous psychometric testing (Streiner and Norman 1995). Essentially, the measure must be valid, reliable and sensitive. Validity is how well the instrument measures what it purports to measure. Reliability is concerned with whether the same measurement can be obtained on other occasions and concerns the amount of error inherent in any measurement. Sensitivity is concerned with how sensitive the measure is to detecting small, or clinically relevant, changes in health/QOL. This is important for monitoring benefits of treatment.

Types of QOL measure

There is no 'gold standard' for measuring QOL and a large number of instruments have been developed for different purposes (Brooks 1995).

- Generic instruments cover a broad range of QOL domains in a single instrument. Their chief advantage is in facilitating comparisons among different disease groups
- Disease-specific instruments reduce patient burden by including only relevant items for a particular illness but their main disadvantage is the lack of comparability of results with those from other disease groups
- Health profiles provide separate scores for each of the dimensions of QOL
- Health indexes are a type of generic instrument, giving a single summary score, usually from 0 (death) to 1 (perfect health). A further category, developed within the economic tradition, is that of utility measures (Spiegelhalter et al 1992; Fenny et al 1996)

A common recommendation is to use both specific and generic measures in any study assessing QOL (Fletcher et al 1992).

Because of the complex issues involved in the assessment of QOL in dementia,

three broad methods have been developed:

- Direct observation of the patient's behaviour
- Caregiver informed: obtaining information on QOL of the patient from the caregiver alone
- Patient rated: scales that ask the patient to rate their own QOL

It has been recommended that the assessment of QOL in dementia should include disease-specific instruments, that take account of staging of the disease (Rockwood and Wilcock 1996) and that the views and values of each patient and their family or other carers should be included (Rockwood and Wilcock 1996; Rabins and Kasper 1997).

QOL measures used in dementia research

The Schedule for the Evaluation of Individual Quality of Life (SEIQOL)

Patients with dementia were asked to rate their own QOL using an individualized measure called the Schedule for the Evaluation of Individual Quality of Life (SEIQOL). With this approach, devised from a technique known as judgement analysis, patients rate their level of functioning in five self-nominated facets of life and then indicate the relative weight or importance they attach to each. The procedure is complex, however, and in this study only six of the 20 patients completed the full assessment (Coen et al 1993). Although the SEIQOL has been validated in a number of patient groups, the results of this study suggest that it may only be of use in patients with very mild dementia.

The Quality of Life Assessment Schedule (QOLAS)

The Quality of Life Assessment Schedule (QOLAS) is another method which is subject-driven, ie, personally tailored to each individual patient. The QOLAS is based on existing psychological theories and methods: Personal Construct Theory and the Repertory Grid Technique (RGT). The RGT was initially developed as a generic tool to assess the QOL of patients with neurological disorders, particularly epilepsy (Kendrick and Trimble 1994). The full Repertory Grid Technique was lengthy and cumbersome and it was deemed desirable to streamline the method. The brief version has been used in a study of patients with epilepsy (Selai and Trimble 1998), and more recently

has been modified for use in patients with dementia. In the dementia study, evidence of construct validity was obtained by looking at correlations with the MMSE and with a number of other disease-specific and generic instruments. Full testing of the psychometric properties of the modified version is ongoing.

Quality of Life-AD (QOL-AD)

The Quality of Life-AD (QOL-AD) obtains a rating of the patient's QOL from both the patient and the caregiver (Logsdon 1996). The scale is based on a literature review on quality of life in older adults and on the assessment of QOL in other chronically ill populations. It has 13 items covering physical health, energy, mood, living situation, memory, family, marriage, friends, chores, fun, money, self and life as a whole. Each of the items are rated as poor, fair, good or excellent. The briefness of the scale, and its self-report format incorporating both patient and caregiver ratings makes it attractive for use in clinical trials. Early validation studies suggest it is a reliable and valid instrument.

Dementia QOL (DQOL)

This recently developed instrument has been designed for direct respondent assessment in cognitively impaired populations (Brod et al 1996). The DQOL was originally a 96-item interview including aspects of physical functioning, daily activities, discretionary activities, mobility, social well-being, interaction capacity, bodily well-being, psychological well-being, sense of aesthetics, and overall quality of life. Some aspects were deleted and the current 56-item version takes approximately 15–20 min to complete. Evidence of the reliability and the validity of a number of the DQOL scales has been obtained.

The Community Dementia QOL Profile (CDQLP)

This is a disease-specific, self-administered instrument which consists of two sections. Part I is a measure of the patient's quality of life assessed by their carer as a proxy and part II is a measure of the carer's own QOL and stress (Salek et al 1996). This is a 33-item instrument with four dimensions including thinking and behaviour, family and social life, physical activities and other aspects of daily living. Construct validation has been performed by looking at correlation with the MMSE. Full testing of the psychometric properties of the scale is ongoing.

Blau QOL Scale

The Blau QOL scale, based on a 'social indicators' approach, assesses QOL in 10 areas relating to working, leisure, eating, sleeping, social contact, earning, parenting, loving, environment and self-acceptance (Blau 1977). It is completed by the patient or, in the institutional setting, by a proxy. The items emerged from interviews with patients in individual and group psychotherapy. The instrument is not specific to dementia and extends beyond ADL to social relationships and subjective states. A subset of seven of these items were rated by the patient in a clinical trial of donepezil (Rogers et al 1998). The areas chosen covered relationships, eating and sleeping, and social and leisure activity. There is no evidence, however, that this generic scale was previously validated for use in dementia and the method of scoring, using a visual analogue scale, would be a problem for patients with apraxia or significant visuo-perceptual difficulties.

The York Scale

In a study looking at long-term psychiatric patients in the community, including 100 patients with senile dementia (Jones et al 1986), QOL was assessed using a scale devised for the study based on Maslow's hierarchy of needs (see **Table 5.2**). The authors reported that the scale required further development. In this study few patients were capable of answering questions and most of the information came from proxies, although often even professional staff were uncertain in their replies.

Cognitively Impaired Life Quality Scale (CILQ)

Based on a series of focus groups with nursing staff, an instrument to measure the QOL of profoundly impaired patients through nursing caregivers' eyes was developed (DeLetter et al 1995). A 29-item version of the Cognitively Impaired Life Quality Scale (CILQ) scale and shortened, 14-item version of the scale are being developed. The 14-item version for clinical use has five categories comprising social interaction, basic physical care, appearance to others, nutrition/hydration and pain/comfort. Full psychometric testing is ongoing.

Byrne–MacLean QOL index

This is a 56-item scale reflecting six categories of concern identified by residents of nursing homes including 'niceness' (patient perception of staff),

worry, care and comfort, choice, physical environment and social needs (Byrne and MacLean 1997). Although the scale developers have described it as a QOL instrument, it perhaps assesses quality of care rather than quality of life.

Other instruments used in dementia

A number of other instruments have been used to assess some aspect of QOL in dementia although they were not specifically designed for this purpose. These have included both generic instruments as yet unvalidated for use in patients with dementia and dementia-specific measures which tap some component of well-being but which might not be technically regarded as a QOL measure (Walker et al 1998).

Observational techniques

A number of techniques have been developed based on observational methods where behaviour of patients is rated by researchers or nursing staff usually for discrete periods of 10 or 15 min. Events, activities or social interactions are coded according to a specified protocol. These include: The Philadelphia Geriatric Center Affect Rating Scale (Lawton 1994); the Short Observation Method (SOM) (MacDonald et al 1985); the Quality of Interactions Schedule (QUIS) (Dean et al 1993) and Dementia Care Mapping (Bredin et al 1995).

There are two other observational techniques still in development by Beck and Volicer & Hurley (Whitehouse et al, 1998; Whitehouse 1998).

Evaluation of current therapies

A review in 1995 of QOL measures used in anti-dementia drug trials for Alzheimer's disease, found that few treatments were assessed for their effect on QOL, and that most instruments used at that time to assess QOL in anti-dementia drug trials had not been adequately validated in patients with Alzheimer's disease (Howard and Rockwood 1995).

The International Working Group recently published a position paper on the harmonization of dementia drug guidelines (Whitehouse et al 1997). This emphasizes the importance of quality of life as an outcome measure when considering the future of international drug development for individuals affected by Alzheimer's disease and other dementias.

Quality of life was assessed in a clinical trial of donepezil, although the scale used (Blau 1977) is a generic scale and probably unsuitable for the task. It is therefore not surprising that results were very variable, and no treatment effect could be discerned (Rogers et al 1998).

The Progressive Deterioration Scale (PDS) (DeJong et al 1989) was used as a measure of QOL, along with the Instrumental Activities of Daily Living (IADL) assessment (Lawton and Brady 1969) and the Physical Self Maintenance Scale (PSMS) (Lawton and Brady 1969) as secondary measures, in clinical trials of tacrine (Davis et al 1992; Farlow et al 1992; Knapp et al 1994). Although the tacrine group did better on some of the QOL scores it can be questioned whether any of these measures comprehensively assesses QOL, as opposed to activities of daily living.

Cost-utility analysis

Cost-utility analysis is a technique that uses the Quality Adjusted Life Year (QALY) as an outcome measure. For its calculation, the QALY requires well-being or QOL to be expressed as a single index score. The Quality of

Well-being scale (QWB) is a utility-weighted measure of health-related quality of life that can be used in clinical trials and cost-utility analyses. Evidence has recently been reported for the validity of the QWB in patients with Alzheimer's disease (Kerner et al 1998).

Future developments

The assessment of QOL in dementia raises a large number of methodological considerations and researchers are attempting to meet the challenge in a variety of ways. Quality of life data are a relevant measure of outcome of therapy and an important basis for economic decisions. Several instruments are in development and the psychometric testing of these is ongoing. We have yet to see a fully validated instrument, which comprehensively assesses QOL, and that can discern the effects of any anti-dementia treatment.

Acknowledgements

Richard Harvey is supported by an Alzheimer's Disease Society Research Fellowship. Caroline Selai acknowledges the support of the Raymond Way Neuropsychiatry Research Fund.

References

Blau TH (1977) Quality of life, social indicators, and criteria of change. *Prof Psychol* **11**:464–73.

Bredin K, Kitwood T, Wattis J (1995) Decline in quality of life for patients with severe dementia following a ward merger. *Int J Geriatr Psychiat* **10**:967–73.

Brod M, Stewart AL (1994) Quality of life of persons with dementia: a theoretical framework. *Gerontologist* **34**:47.

Brod M, Stewart A, Sands L et al (1996) The dementia quality of life rating scale (D-QOL). *Gerontologist* **36**(special issue 1):257.

Brooks RG (1995) *Health Status Measurement: A Perspective on Change.* Macmillian Press, Basingstoke, UK.

Byrne H, Maclean D (1997) Quality of life: perceptions of residential care. *Int J Nurse Pract* **3**:21–8.

Coen R, O'Mahoney D, O'Boyle C et al (1993) Measuring the quality of life of dementia patients using the schedule for the evaluation of individual quality of life. Special issue: psychologial aspects of ageing: well-being and vulnerability. *Irish J Psychol* **14**:154–63.

Davis KL, Thal LJ, Gamzu ER et al (1992) A double-blind, placebo-controlled multicenter study of tacrine for Alzheimer's disease. *N Engl J Med* **327**:1253–59.

Dean R, Proudfoot R, Lindesay J (1993) The Quality of Interactions Schedule (QUIS): development, reliability and use in the evaluation of two domus units. *Int J Geriatr Psychiat* **8**:819–26.

Dejong R, Osterlund OW, Roy GW (1989) Measurement of quality of life changes in patients with Alzheimer's disease. *Clin Ther* **11**:545–54.

DeLetter MC, Tully CL, Wilson JF, Rich EC (1995) Nursing staff perceptions of quality of life of cognitively impaired elders: instrumental development. *J Appl Gerontol* **4**:426–43.

Farlow M, Gracon SI, Hershey LA et al (1992) A controlled trial of tacrine in Alzheimer's disease. *JAMA* **268**:2523–29.

Fenny DH, Torrance GW, Labelle R (1996) Integrating economic evaluations and quality of life assessments. In: Spilker B (ed) *Quality of Life and Pharmacoeconomics In Clinical Trials*. Lippincott-Raven, Philadelphia.

Fitzpatrick R, Fletcher A, Gore S et al (1992) Quality of life measures in health care. I: applications and issues in assessment. *BMJ* **305**:1074–7.

Fletcher AE, Gore SM, Spiegelhalter DJ et al (1992) Quality of life measures in health

care. II: design, analysis and interpretation. *BMJ* **305**:1145–48.

Howard K, Rockwood K (1995) Quality of life in Alzheimer's disease: a review. *Dementia* **6**:113–6.

Jones K, Robinson M, Golightley M (1986) Long-term psychiatric patients in the community. *Br J Psychiatry* **149**:537–40.

Kelly CA, Harvey RJ, Cayton H (1997) Drug treatments for Alzheimer's disease. *BMJ* **314**:693–4.

Kendrick AM, Trimble MR (1994) Repertory grid in the assessment of quality of life in patients with epilepsy: The quality of life assessment schedule. In: Trimble MR, Dodson WE (eds) *Epilepsy and Quality of Life*. Raven, Philadelphia.

Kerner DN, Paterson TK, Grant, Kaplan RM (1998) Validity of the quality of well-being scale for patients with Alzheimer's disease. *J Aging Health* **10**:44–61.

Knapp MJ, Knopman DS, Solomon PR et al (1994) A 30-week randomised controlled trial of high-dose tacrine in patients with Alzheimer's disease. *JAMA* **271**:985–91.

Lawton MP (1994) Quality of life in Alzheimer disease. *Alzheimer Dis Assoc Disord* **8**(Suppl 3):138–50.

Lawton MP (1997) Assessing quality of life

in Alzheimer disease research. *Alzheimer Dis Assoc Disord* **11**(Suppl 6):91–9.

Lawton MP, Brody EM (1969) Assessment of older people: self-maintaining and instrumental activities of daily living. *Gerontologist* **9**:176–86.

Logsdon RG (1996) Quality of life in Alzheimer's disease: implications for research *Gerontologist* **36**(Special Issue 1):278.

MacDonald AJD, Craig TKJ, Warner LAR (1985) The development of a short observation method for the study of activity and contacts of old people in residential settings. *Psychol Med* **15**:167–72.

Rabins PV, Kasper JD (1997) Measuring quality of life in dementia: conceptual and practical issues. *Alzheimer Dis Assoc Disord* **11**(Suppl 6):100–4.

Revicki DA (1996) Relationship of pharmacoeconomics and health-related quality of life. In: Spilker B (ed) *Quality of Life and Pharmacoeconomics In Clinical Trials.* Lippincott-Raven, Philadelphia.

Rockwood K, Wilcock GK (1996) Quality of life. In: Gauthier S (ed) *Clinical Diagnosis and Management of Alzheimers Disease* Martin Dunitz, London: 279–90.

Rogers SL, Farlow MR, Doody RS, Mohs R, Friedhoff LT and the Donepezil Study Group (1998) A 24-week, double-blind, placebo-controlled trial of donepezil in patients with Alzheimer's disease. *Neurology* **50**:136–45.

Salek MS, Schwartzberg E, Bayer AJ (1996) Evaluating health-related quality of life in patients with dementia: development of a proxy self-administered questionnaire (abstract). *Pharm World Sci* **18**(5 Suppl A)6.

Selai CE, Trimble MR (1998) Adjunctive therapy in epilepsy with new antiepileptic drugs: is it of any value? *Seizure* **7**:417–8.

Spiegelhalter DJ, Gore SM, Fitzpatrick R et al (1992) Quality of life measures in health care. III: resource allocation. *BMJ* **305**:1205–9.

Stewart AL, Sherbourne CD, Brod M (1996) Measuring health-related quality of life in older and demented populations. In: Spilker B (ed) *Quality of Life and Pharmacoeconomics In Clinical Trials.* Lippincott-Raven, Philadelphia.

Streiner DL, Norman GR (1995) *Health Measurement Scales: A Practical Guide to Their Development and Use.* 2nd edn. Oxford University Press, Oxford.

Walker MD, Salek SS, Bayer AJ (1998) A review of quality of life in Alzheimer's disease. Part 1: issues in assessing disease impact. *PharmacoEconomics* **14**:499–530.

Whitehouse PJ (1998) Quality of life in dementia. In: Wimo A, Jonsson G, Karlsson G, Winblad B (eds) *Health Economics and Dementia*. John Whiley, Chichester, 403–17.

Whitehouse PJ, Orgogozo J-M, Becker RE et al (1997) Quality of life assessment in dementia drug development. Position paper from the International Working Group on Harmonization of Dementia Drug Guidelines. *Alzheimer Dis Assoc Disord* **11**(Suppl 3):56–60.

Whitehouse PJ, Winblad B, Shostak D et al (1998) 1st International Pharmacoeconomic Conference on Alzheimer's Disease: report and summary. *Alzheimer Dis Assoc Disord* **12**:266–80.

Caregiver burden

6

As has been described in previous chapters the progressive nature of Alzheimer's disease (AD) results in sufferers becoming more and more dependent on the caregiver. This person is usually a close relative, rather than a professional carer, and as a result of the ageing of our population we are witnessing an ever-increasing number of unpaid caregivers of the frail and ill elderly.

Caring for someone with AD is particularly burdensome and AD has been described as an illness of two people — the sufferer and the carer. Most AD sufferers live in the community and their carers are central to their management, giving consistent care and often providing professionals with important information about the patient's symptoms. It has been estimated that the annual cost to society for caring for a person with dementia in the home is half that for an institutionalized patient so, quite apart from the necessity in the absence of alternative provisions, there are substantial financial savings to the health care system of informal caregiving. The wellbeing of these caregivers is therefore extremely important for the continuing care of AD patients in the community.

Effects of caregiving

There have been a number of studies on the effects of being a caregiver looking at the physical, psychological and social outcomes in the carer and how the different facets of the patient's illness have been linked to caregiver morbidity. Much of the caregiver literature has focused on the concept of caregiver burden (CGB), which has been operationalized in a number of ways. Broadly speaking CGB can be defined as the consequence for carers of the practical and emotional demands that result from caregiving. It is a complex process involving developmental and cultural factors in addition to the stress of caring. Also influential are the carers gender, their coping style, social network and the level of intimacy with the dependent. The impact of caring has been found to persist even after the patient has been institutionalized and so is not limited to only those carers in the community.

> **Caregiver Burden**
> *(objective burden and perceived stress)*
>
> *Caregiver burden refers to 'the physical, psychological or emotional, social and financial problems that can be experienced by family members caring for impaired older adults'. (George and Gwyther 1986)*

Recent reviews of the literature have tended to focus on psychiatric symptomatology in carers, especially depression. The patient–caregiver relationship is a complicated one and a number of different outcomes can result. Pearlin et al (1990) conceptualized the caregiver stress paradigm which looked at primary stressors including the degree of impairment of the patient and the expression of disease symptoms, and the secondary stressors which result as an indirect effect of caregiving, eg, constriction of social life, loss of self and in younger carers the job–caregiving conflict. Life for the caregiver becomes dominated by caring for the patient leaving little time for considering his or her own needs. These conflicts can cause resentment, guilt and anger and have an effect on

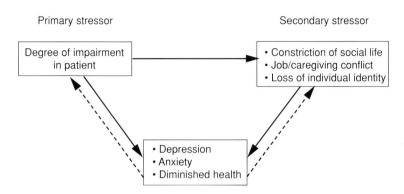

Figure 6.1
Stress paradigm

the caregiver's health. Poor health in the caregiver can further confound the secondary stressors which can have a negative effect on the patient, thus creating a vicious cycle (**Figure 6.1**).

Measurement of caregiver burden

There are no gold standards for the measurement of caregiver burden and many studies developed their own individual scales which have then not been used again. However, there are key themes which appear to be universal to the various scales, these include:

- *Overall distress and strain*
- *Financial concerns*
- *Isolation and lack of family support*
- *Physical and/or emotional health*
- *Self esteem and self worth*
- *Emotional stress, ie, hostility, grief, guilt, resentment*

Scales which are more commonly used to measure CGB which have been shown to be sensitive, specific and reliable are listed in **Figure 6.2.** Assessment of caregiver burden is an independent parameter when looking

---

Screen for Caregiver Burden *(Vitiliano 1991)*
Measures distress related to patient impairment (cognition, function, impairment), disruptions in family and social life, and caregiver affective responses.

Twenty-five item questionnaire, eg, He does not recognize me/Constantly asks the same questions/Been embarrassed etc.

Two scores: Subjective — Severity of distress experienced by caregiver. Objective — The number of distressing experiences.

Poulshock & Deimling Cognitive Subscale *(Poulshock et al 1984)*
Eight-item questionnaire, eg, he has been confused, wandered, seen things etc.

Measures the distress caused specifically by the different aspects of the cognitive impairment of the patient.

Abridged Relative Stress Scale *(Greene et al 1982; Kaufer et al 1998)*
Assesses the overall psychological impact on the caregiver to the caregiving situation.

Ten-item questionnaire, eg, Have you been cross in anyway with the patient/Felt you needed a break etc.

Figure 6.2
Caregiver burden scales

at improvement in AD and should be used when treatments for AD are being assessed.

Impact of patient impairments on caregiver

Alzheimer's disease can be seen to have four symptomatic domains that all impact on the carer in differing proportions (**Figure 6.3**).

Neuropsychiatric symptoms

The majority of research has found a strong correlation with CGB and this heterogeneous group of symptoms, a much stronger correlation in fact than

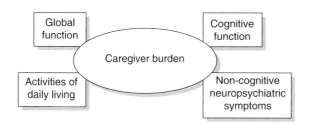

Figure 6.3
Four domains of Alzheimer's disease

with cognitive impairment or even activities of daily life. They consist of:

- *Psychotic symptoms*
  Delusions
  Hallucinations
- *Depressive features*
  Sadness
  Lack of interest
  Apathy/indifference
- *Behaviour disorders*
  Aggression/agitation
  Irritability
  Wandering

In particular, deficits of behaviour (withdrawal and apathy) are more closely related to increased CGB than excesses of behaviour (hoarding, sleep disturbances). Certain aspects of disturbed behaviour such as aggression, mood changes and withdrawal are closely related to negative changes in the caregivers' feeling towards the patient resulting in a disruption of the previous affectionate relationship.

Cognitive function

The relationship between cognitive impairment and CGB is more complex and would appear to depend on the degree of impairment. Carers report more stress in the very early stages of the dementia than when memory impairment is more advanced.

Activities of daily living

Activities of daily living (ADLs), eg, self care, managing finances etc, have not been found to have a significant relationship with CGB. One study did find a link between ADL limitations and burden in female carers but not in males (Harper and Lund 1990).

Global effect of CGB on the carer

Carer stress is dependent on a number of factors including gender, relationship of the carer to the patient and the carer's coping styles. Caregiver burden is similar in males and females but men are less likely to discuss their problems. Areas of carer well-being that are most sensitive to the burden of being a carer are:

- Mental health
- Physical health
- Social activity restrictions

Psychological distress of carers as measured on the General Health Questionnaire (GHQ) is closely associated with patient psychopathology; this is consistent with stress in caregiving in other disorders such as cancer. Again behaviour disturbances such as night time wandering, incontinence and immobility were significantly correlated with increased burden.

Depression is frequently seen in carers and some studies quote prevalences of nearly 50%. Carer stress has been found to be a contributing factor towards the increased rate of suicide in the elderly population. Depression is more common in female carers of patients with dementia and there is a strong positive relationship between caregiver depression and aspects of non-cognitive disturbance in patients. Educational interventions which increase the carer's knowledge about dementia appear to offer some protection against depression but may increase levels of anxiety. Active practical coping strategies with the carer taking a firm approach in directing behaviour and being flexible in their daily routines appears to be associated with less depression in the carer.

Only a small number of studies have looked at the physical health of the carer as an outcome of CGB. There is some evidence to suggest that labour intensive ADL limitations are linked to physical ill health but further support for this relationship is needed. Caregivers are at greater risk of social isolation for a variety of reasons. They have the difficulty of leaving the dependent alone, whilst disruptive behaviours, ADL limitations and poor physical self-maintenance are more likely to stop carers' normal social participation.

Implications for management

With the current emphasis on community care, and with the increasing pressures on the health care system, caregivers need to be supported and treated as well as the patient with dementia. Although the needs vary for each individual, carers frequently request help in the following areas:

- *Active treatment for troublesome symptoms*
- *Support from skilled medical staff*
- *Acknowledgement of their burden*
- *Reassurance of continuing professional support*
- *Disease/treatment information*
- *Control over their situation*
- *Choice of care options*

Key Points

- *Non-cognitive features of AD are stressful for carers and are strong predictors of CGB.*

- *Treating depression and behavioural disturbances will not only help patient but reduce carer burden.*

- *Cognitive impairment is associated with CGB in the mild to moderate stages of dementia but diminishes as the illness progresses.*

- *Caregiver burden continues even after the patient is institutionalized.*

- *Good informal support and increased knowledge of the illness reduce caregiver burden.*

Carers provide consistent care for the patient and play a large part in relieving the financial strain on the health care services by preventing or delaying the need for institutionalization (**Figure 6.4**).

Clearly the ideal solution would be to cure the patient. Current treatments fall far short of this but can still impact on and reduce carer burden; hitherto treatment of troublesome symptoms was based purely on the use of tranquilizers, antidepressants and hypnotics. However, these treatments can have troublesome side effects of sedation or worsening confusion. The new rational treatments, based on cholinesterase inhibition have been shown not only to reduce neuropsychiatric symptoms and improve cognition in the patient but also to reduce carer burden. In one study there was a marked decrease in time spent caring by the carers of

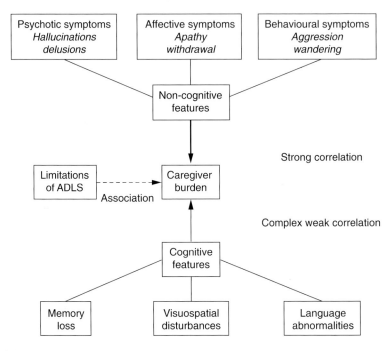

Figure 6.4
Impact of Alzheimer's disease on caregiver

patients taking Velnacrine compared with placebo. A large double-blind study showed significant reductions in three different measures of carer burden in carers of patients taking Metrifonate compared with those on placebo. It seems likely therefore that whilst simple support will help, real reductions in carer burden will only occur as the patient and their troublesome symptoms are treated. By identifying specific impairments which are likely to increase caregiver burden, future interventions can be tailored to reduce both patient and carer distress.

References

Clipp EC, Moore MJ (1995) Caregiver time use: an outcome measure in clinical trial research on Alzheimer's disease. *Clin Pharmacol Ther* **58**:228–36.

Coen RF, Swanwick GR, O'Boyle CA et al (1997) Behaviour disturbance and other predictors of carer burden in Alzheimer's disease. *Int J Geriatr Psychiatry* **12**:331–6.

Donaldson C, Tarrier N, Burns A (1997) The impact of the symptoms of dementia on caregivers. *Br J Psychiatry* **170**:62–8.

George LK, Gwyther LP (1986) Caregiver well-being: a multidimensional examination of family caregivers of demented adults. *Gerontologist* **26**:253–9.

Greene JG, Smith R, Timbury GG (1982) Measuring behavioural disturbance of elderly demented patients in the community and its effects on relatives: a factor analytic study. *Age and Ageing* **11**:121–6.

Harper S, Lund DA (1990) Wives, husbands and daughters caring for institutionalized and noninstitutionalized dementia patients: toward a model of caregiver burden. *Int J Aging Hum Dev* **30**:241–62.

Kaufer DI, Cummings JL, Christine D et al (1998) Assessing the impact of neuropsychiatric symptoms in Alzheimer's disease: the Neuropsychiatric Inventory in Caregiver Distress Scale. *J Am Geriatr Soc* **46**:210–15.

Pearlin LI, Mullan JT, Semple SJ, Skaff MM (1990) Caregiver and the stress process: an overview of concepts and their measures. *Gerontologist* **30**:583–94.

Poulshock SW, Deimling GT (1984) Families caring for elders in residence: issues in the measurement of burden. *J Gerontol* **39**:230–9.

Shikiar R, Shakespeare A, Sagnier P et al (1998) The impact on caregivers of Metrifonate Therapy administered to patients with Alzheimer's disease: results from a clinical trial. In press.

Vitiliano PP, Young HM, Russo J (1991) Burden: a review of measures used among caregivers of individuals with dementia. *Gerontologist* **31**:67–75.

Index

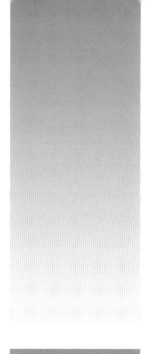

activities of daily living (ADLs) 28
  assessment
    objectives 29-30
    as outcome measure 33
    tools 30-1
  changes in AD 27-9
    impact on caregiver 67, 68
  instrumental 28
  self-care 28
Activities of Daily Living Situational Test 30
aggression, treatment 43
agitation 38, 39, 41-2
  treatment 43, 44, 45, 47
Alzheimer's Disease Assessment Scale (ADAS-COG) 6, 7
  treatment evaluation 8-11
Alzheimer's disease co-operative study – clinical global
    impression of change (ADCS-CGIC) 20, 21, 22
anti-dementia drugs evaluation
  cognitive effects 8-11
  global function assessment 15-25
    current therapies 22-3
  quality of life measures 58-9
antidepressants 43, 46-7
  tricyclic 43, 47
antioxidant therapies 47-8
antipsychotics 43, 45-6, 47
anxiety 38, 39, 40
  treatment 43, 44, 45, 47

anxiolytics 43, 47
apathy 38, 39
 treatment 44, 45

BEHAVE-AD 41, 42
Behavioral Rating Scale for Dementia 41,
 42
behavioural changes see
 neuropsychiatric symptoms
benzodiazepines 47
beta-blockers 43
Blau QOL Scale 56
Blessed Information, Memory,
 Concentration Test (BIMC) 5, 6
Bristol Activities of Daily Living Scale
 30-1
buspirone 43
Byrne-MacLean QOL index 57

Cambridge Cognitive Examination
 (CAMCOG) 6, 7
CANTAB 11
carbamazepine 43, 47
caregivers 632-4
 burden on 64-5
  lightening of 45, 69-70
  measurement 65-6
 impact of patient impairments 37,
  44-5, 66-8, 70
 management of functional decline 32
 support for 45, 69
CGIS/C (clinical global impression of
 severity/change) 18
cholinesterase inhibitors 33, 45, 48, 69
CIBIC-plus 20-1, 22
 Sandoz/New York University 20, 21,
  22
CIBIS/C (clinicians interview-based
 impression of severity/change)
 18-19
 Parke-Davis 19-20, 21
citalopram 43, 47
Clinical Dementia Rating (CDR) 17-18, 19
COGDRAS 11

cognitive decline 1-2
 criteria 2
 functional decline and 29
 impact on caregiver 67
 rate of 4
cognitive testing/assessment
 objectives 2-4
 screening programmes 3, 5-6
 symptoms to be assessed 4-5
 tools/procedures 5-8
  floor to ceiling effects 8, 11
  treatment evaluation 8-11
Cognitively Impaired Life Quality Scale
 (CILQ) 57
Cohen-Mansfield Agitation Inventory 41,
 42
Community Demential QOL Profile
 (CDQLP) 56
computer-aided assessment of cognitive
 function 11
Cornell Scale for Depression in
 Dementia 42
cost-utility analysis 58-9

delusions 38, 39
 treatment 44, 45
Dementia Care Mapping 58
dementia with Lewy bodies (DLB) 3
Dementia QOL (DQOL) 55-6
depression 38-40, 42
 caregivers 68
 treatment 43, 45, 46-7
desipramine 43, 47
diagnosis of dementia
 cognitive assessment 3-4, 7
 subtypes 3, 7
Direct Assessment of Function 30
disinhibition 39
 treatment 44, 45
divalproex 43, 47
donepezil
 cognitive impairment 10
 functional decline 33
 global function assessment 22

neuropsychiatric symptoms 45
quality of life effects 58
driving 28, 31
  assessment 31
dysphoria 39, 44

eptastigmine 45
euphoria 39, 44

fluoxetine 43, 47
fluvoxamine 43, 47
fronto-temporal dementia (FTD) 4
Functional Assessment Staging (FAST)
  18, 19, 31
functional decline 27
  assessment 29, 32
  cognitive decline and 29
  management 31-3
  treatment 33
  see also activities of daily living

galantamine, neuropsychiatric symptoms
  45
galanthamine, global outcome
  assessment 23
ginkgo biloba
  cognitive effects 10
  global outcome assessment 23
Global Deterioration Scale (GDS) 18, 19
global function assessment 15-25
  absolute global severity assessments
    16-17
  clinical global measures 18-21
  current therapies 22-3
  disease staging measures 15-16, 17-18,
    19
  future developments 23-4
  objectives 15-17

hallucinations 38, 39
  treatment 44, 45
  visual 45
haloperidol 43, 46
hormonal therapies 49

insomnia 43, 47
Instrumental Activities of Daily Living
  (IADL) 58
Interview for Deterioration in Daily
  Functioning Activities 30
IQ, premorbid, assessment 3
irritability 39, 40
  treatment 44

Kendrick Test Battery 6

lorazepam 43, 47

Mattis Dementia Rating Scale (DRS) 6, 7
memory impairment 1-2
metrifonate 70
  cognitive impairment 10
  functional decline 33
  global outcome assessment 22
  neuropsychiatric symptoms 45, 46
Mini Mental State Examination (MMSE)
  5, 6, 7, 8
misidentification syndromes 40
mood changes 38-40
mood stabilizing agents 43, 47
motor activity, aberrant 39, 40
  treatment 44, 45

National Adult Reading Test (NART) 3
nefazodone 43
neuroleptics see antipsychotics
Neuropsychiatric Inventory 41, 42, 44, 46
neuropsychiatric symptoms 38-40
  assessment
    future developments 48-9
    objectives 37-8
    rating scales 41-2
    syndromic approach 40-1
  impact on caregiver 37, 44-5, 66-7
  treatment
    disease-modifying 47-8
    future developments 48-9
    non-pharmacological 43-5
    pharmacological 42-3

New York University CIBIC-plus (NYU
CIBIC-plus) 20, 21, 22
nonsteroidal anti-inflammatory drugs
(NSAIDs) 47–8
nortriptyline 43, 47

occupational therapist, assessment of
functional impairment 31
oestrogen replacement therapy 49
olanzapine 43, 46
oxazepam 43, 47

Parke–Davis CIBIC 19–20, 21
paroxetine 43, 47
personality changes 40
Philadelphia Geriatric Center Affect
Rating Scale 57
Physical Self Maintenance Scale (PSMS) 58
physostigmine, long-acting 45
picture sign 40
Progressive Deterioration Scale (PDS) 30,
58
propentofylline, global outcome
assessment 23
propranolol 43, 47
psychiatric symptoms see
neuropsychiatric symptoms
psychosis, treatment 43

Quality Adjusted Life Year (QALY) 58
Quality of Interactions Schedule (QUIS) 58
quality of life (QOL)
assessment
future developments 59
measurement instruments 53–8
objectives 51–2
symptoms assessed 52, 53
in treatment evaluation 58–9
definition 51
Quality of Life-AD (QOL-AD) 55
Quality of Life Assessment Schedule
(QOLAS) 55
Quality of Well-being scale (QWB) 58–9
quetiapine 43, 46

rate of progression, cognitive testing 4
Repertory Grid Technique (RGT) 55
risperidone 43, 46
rivastigmine
cognitive impairment 10
functional decline 33
global function assessment 22
neuropsychiatric symptoms 45

Sandoz/New York University CIBIC-plus
20, 21, 22
Schedule for the Evaluation of Individual
Quality of Life (SEIQOL) 54–5
screening, cognitive 3, 5–6
sedative-hypnotics 43, 47
selective serotonin re-uptake inhibitors
43, 47
selegiline 47–8
self-care 28
sertraline 43, 47
Severe Impairment Battery (SIB) 7, 8, 11
severity of impairment, cognitive testing
4, 5–6
Short Observation Method (SOM) 57
stress, caregivers 64–5, 67–8
Syndrome Kurztest (SKT) 5, 6

tacrine
cognitive impairment 10
functional decline 33
neuropsychiatric symptoms 44, 45
quality of life effects 58
temazepam 43, 47
Test for Severe Impairment 8, 11
trazodone 43, 47
tricyclic antidepressants 43, 47

vascular dementia (VaD) 3–4
velnacrine 70
venlafaxine 43, 47
vitamin E 47–8

York Scale 56–7

zolpidem 43, 47